Surgical Reflections

IMAGES IN PAINT AND PROSE

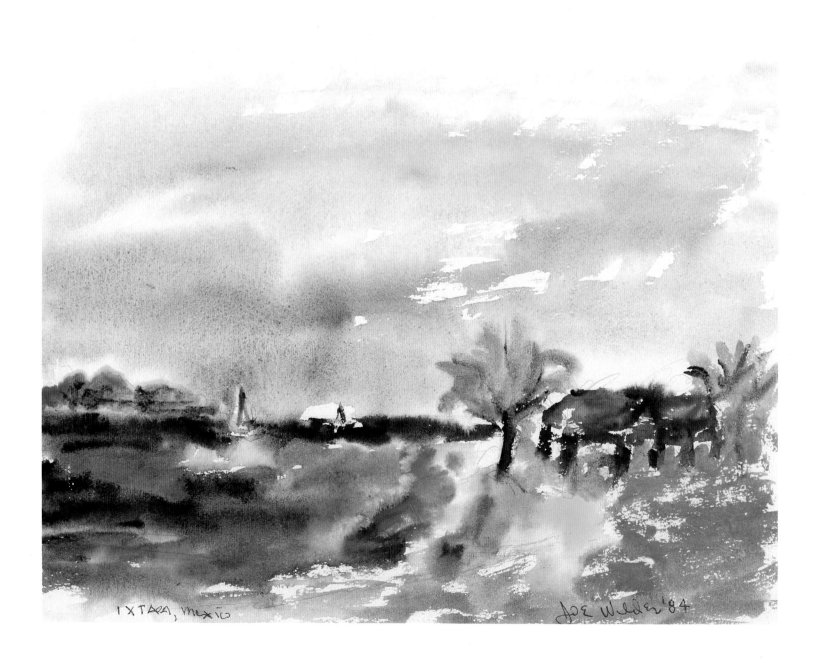

IXTAPA, Mexico   Joe Wilder '84

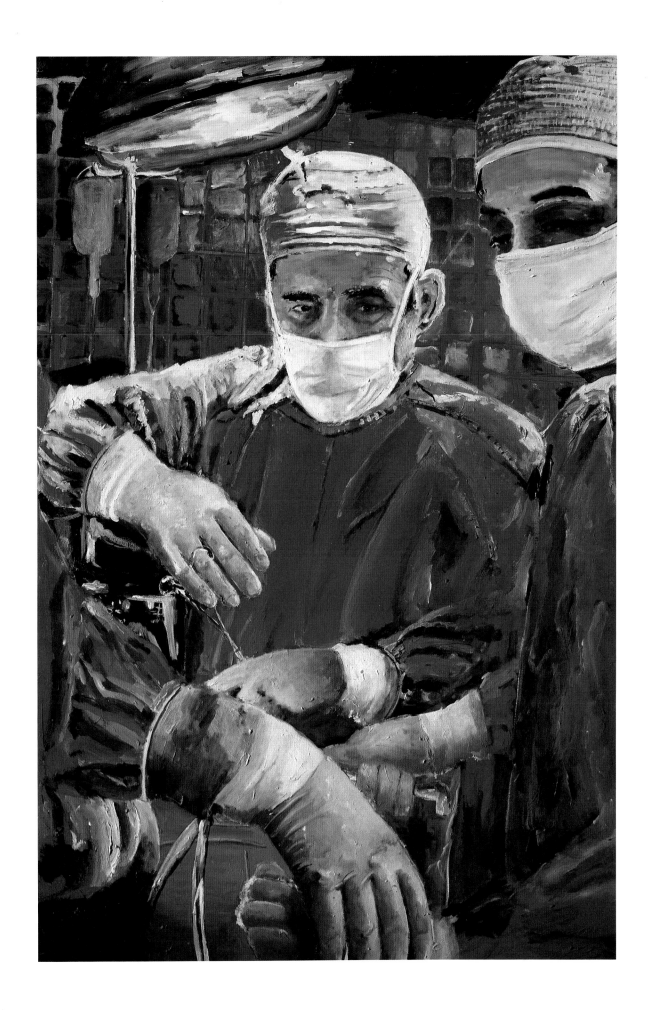

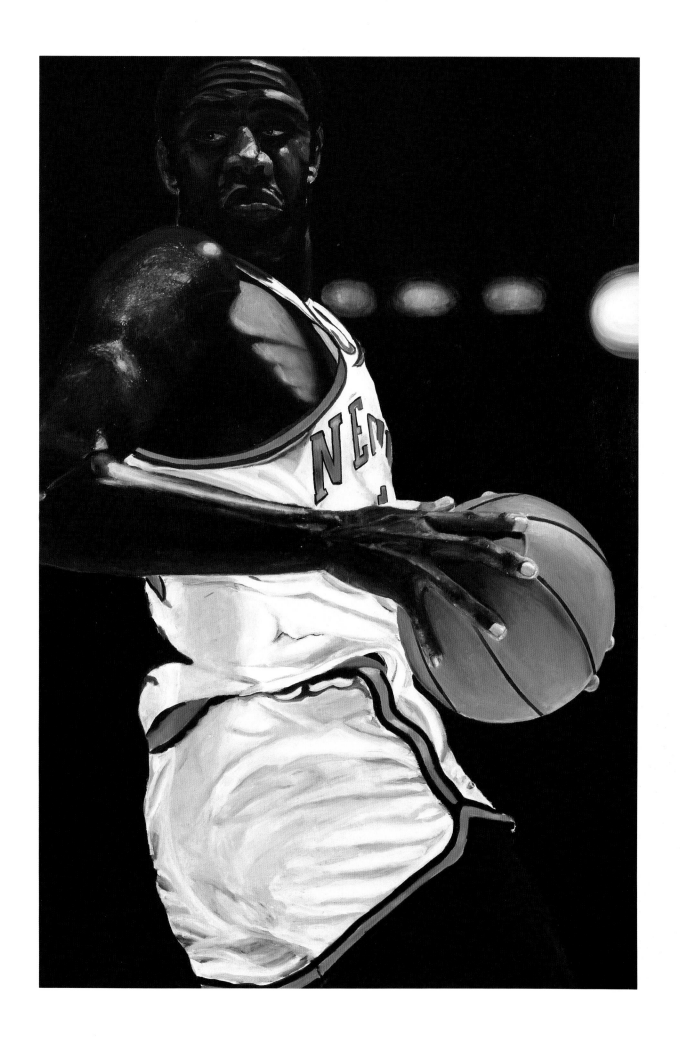

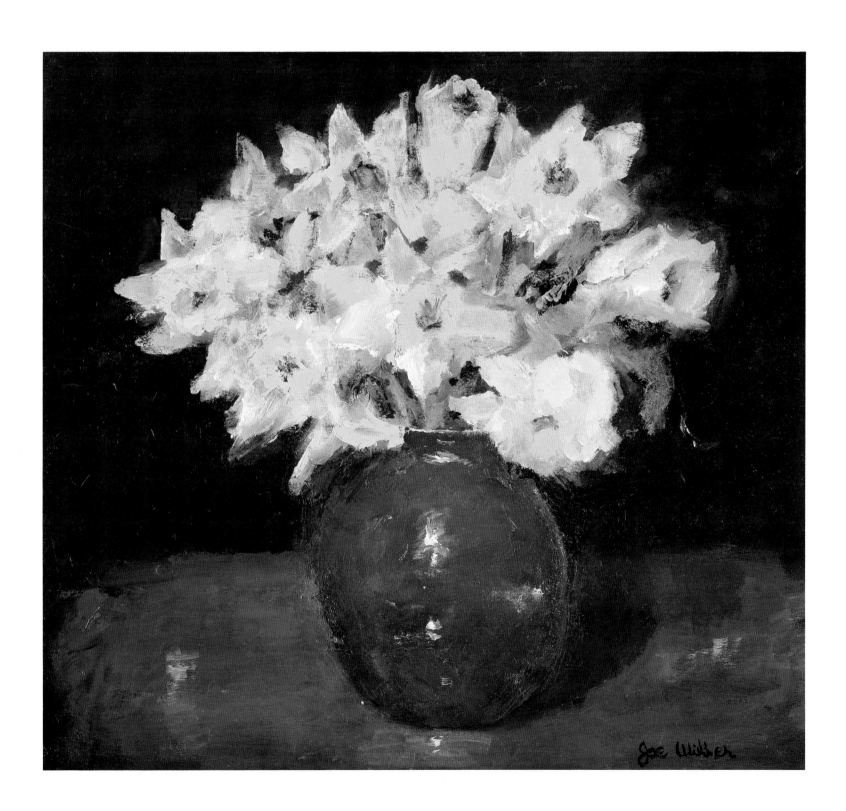

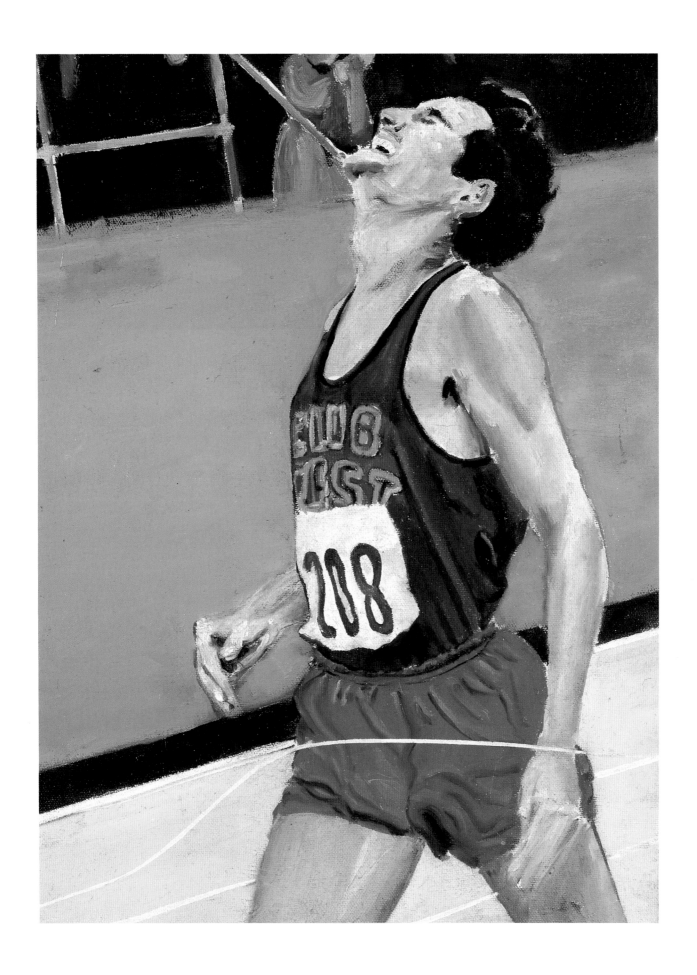

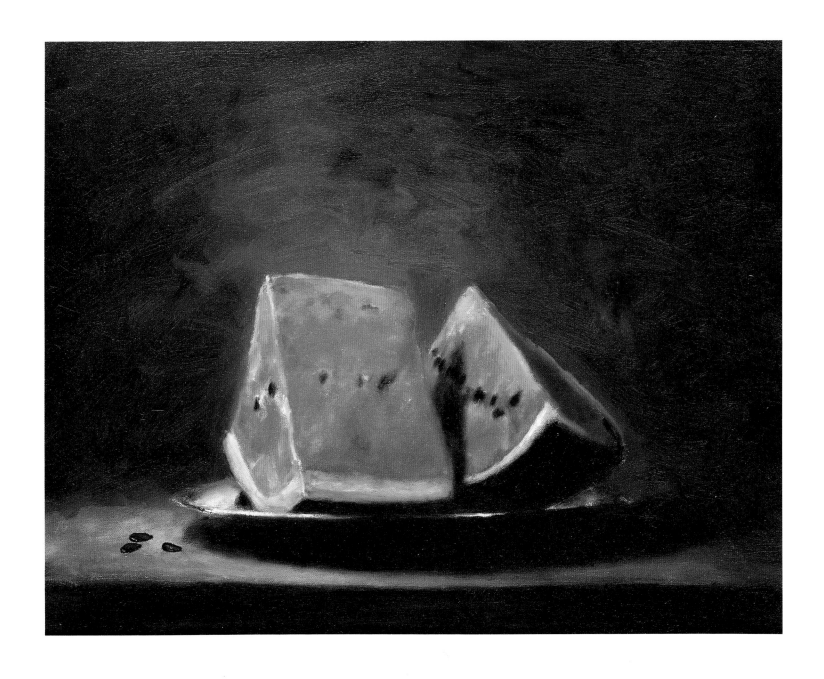

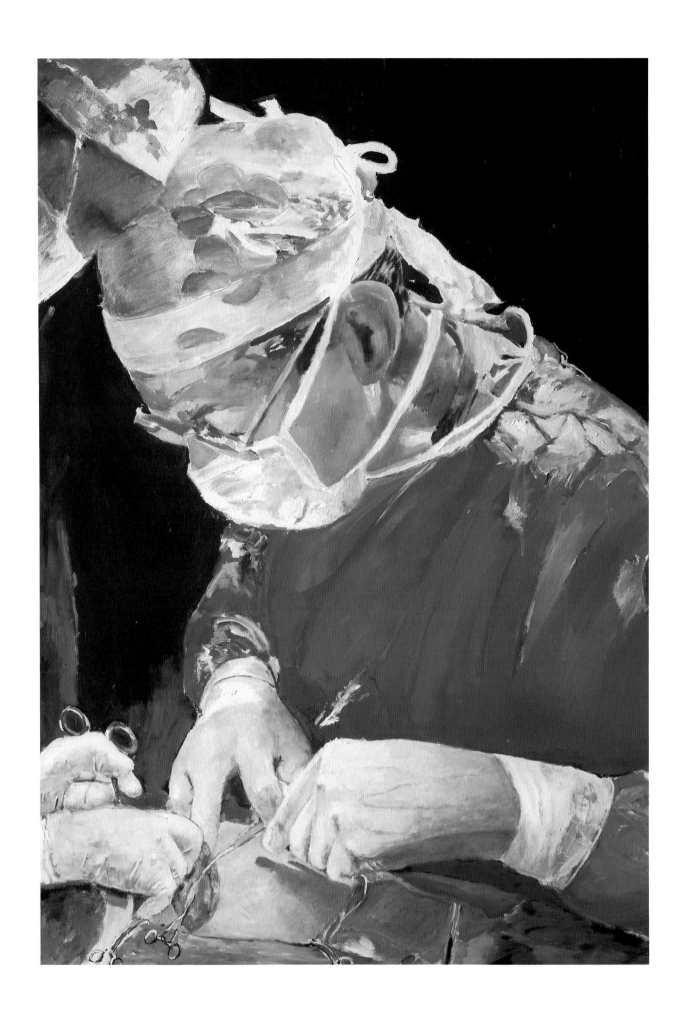

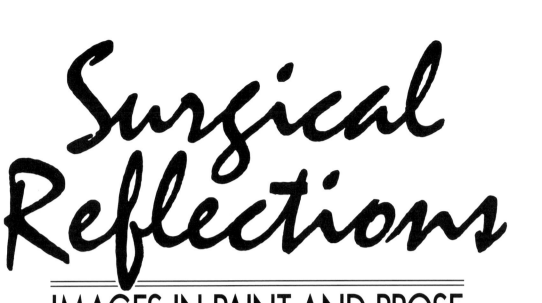

Surgical Reflections

IMAGES IN PAINT AND PROSE

Seymour I. Schwartz, MD

Professor and Chair
Department of Surgery
University of Rochester School of Medicine and Dentistry
Rochester, New York

Joe Wilder, MD

Professor of Surgery, Emeritus
Mount Sinai School of Medicine
New York, New York

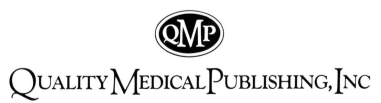

QUALITY MEDICAL PUBLISHING, INC

ST. LOUIS, MISSOURI
1993

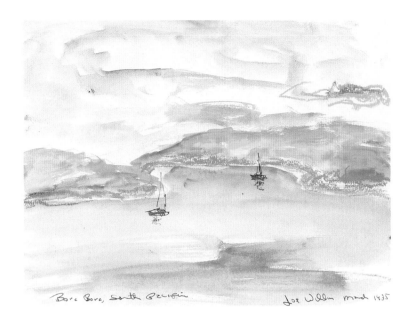

Bora Bora, South Pacific   Joe Wilder march 1935

PUBLISHER Karen Berger
PROJECT EDITOR Suzanne Seeley Wakefield
EDITING ASSISTANT Kathleen J. Jenkins

Designed by Diane Beasley Design, St. Louis, Missouri
Typeset in 12-point Sabon with display in Mistral
by Village Typographers, Inc., Waterloo, Illinois
Produced by Pacific Offset, Ltd., St. Louis, Missouri
Printed in Hong Kong
Printed on 157 GSM Japanese New Age Matte Art Paper
and bound in T-Saifu

Quality Medical Publishing, Inc.
2086 Craigshire Drive
St. Louis, Missouri 63146

LIBRARY OF CONGRESS CATALOGING-IN-PUBLICATION DATA
Schwartz, Seymour I., 1928-
    Surgical reflections : images in paint and prose / Seymour
  I. Schwartz, Joe Wilder.
      p.   cm.
    ISBN 0-942219-48-1
    1. Surgery—Philosophy. 2. Surgery—Miscellanea. 3. Surgery in
  art. I. Wilder, Joe, 1920-   . II. Title.
    [DNLM: 1. Surgery—essays. 2. Surgery—pictorial works.   WO 517
  S399s]
  RD31.5.S36   1993
  617—dc20
  DNLM/DLC
  for Library of Congress   92-49796
                                                          CIP

5 4 3 2 1

Seymour Schwartz, MD, truly epitomizes the essence of the Renaissance man. A noted surgeon, writer, historian, and cartophile, his accomplishments are legion. Dr. Schwartz is Professor and Chair of the Department of Surgery at the University of Rochester. Honored with a Distinguished Service Award by the American College of Surgeons, he is also a regent of that respected organization. Among his other awards and honors are the Markle Scholarship, the prestigious Roswell Park and the Albert D. Kaiser Medals, the University of South Carolina Sesquicentennial Award, honorary membership in many American surgical societies and international colleges of surgeons, and an honorary doctorate from the University of Lund, Sweden. He served as President of the Central Surgical Society and the Society for Clinical Surgery and was Vice-Chairman of the American Board of Surgery. Dr. Schwartz has always been enchanted with the written word and delights in finding *le mot juste:* "The choice of the right word, correctly spelled, in a grammatically acceptable sentence is characteristic of a precise personality," he says, "that which is generally demanded of a surgeon." This passion for writing has been translated into his significant contributions to the surgical literature. He has published more than 200 scientific articles, 200 editorials, and six textbooks and served as Editor-in-Chief of *Contemporary Surgery* and the *Yearbook of Surgery* for two decades. His essays invite the reader to explore the nature of being human and the experience of practicing surgery. The comedy of living stands in sharp relief against the tragedy of dying. He is best known as Editor of *Principles of Surgery,* currently in its sixth edition, the most widely used surgical textbook throughout the world. An abiding interest in the humanities characterizes his writings and peripatetic activities. He is a member of the American Antiquarian Society, the Grolier Club, and the Cosmos Club. As a pathfinder, his interest in the field of cartographic history is a natural corollary. The book *Mapping of America,* which he coauthored, is regarded as the authoritative work on the subject. Dr. Schwartz is currently completing a cartographic history of the battles of the French and Indian War.

Joe Wilder, MD, surgeon, educator, painter, and athlete, is renowned for his vibrant images of athletes in motion and of surgeons at work. His sun-drenched landscapes and seascapes and elegant still lifes have won critical acclaim. Whether rendering the taut trapezius muscles of an Olympic swimmer or the shimmer of light on a tulip petal, Dr. Wilder brings to bear skills perfected as a surgeon: acute powers of observation, knowledge of anatomy, concentration, and a deft, bold hand. As Professor Emeritus of Surgery at Mount Sinai School of Medicine and former Director of Surgery at New York's Hospital of Joint Diseases, he has performed in an arena demanding enormous energy and tenacity. He was a Markle Scholar, awarded by a foundation that seeks out future leaders in medicine. He is the recipient of the Dartmouth Inaugural Medal for Achievement in Art and Medicine and was recently initiated into Phi Beta Kappa. A Dartmouth All American in lacrosse, he has five unbroken sports records to his credit and was inducted into the Lacrosse Hall of Fame. His introduction to the painter's milieu was through his patient and friend, actor Zero Mostel. In Mostel's studio he was mesmerized by the pungent scent of oils and by the rhythm, form, and color in painting the human figure. What followed was a year's orgy of painting, culminating in a return to basics, since his instincts as a surgeon dictated mastery of the fundamentals. For more than three decades Joe Wilder has developed his unique style in a variety of media and subjects, from his deeply pigmented and dynamic works in oil and acrylics to his spritely and spontaneous watercolors. *The New York Times* has hailed him as "a Renaissance man"; his images have also appeared on many covers of the *Journal of the American Medical Association* and *Contemporary Surgery.* He is the author of *Atlas of Surgery* and of an art book, *Athletes: The Paintings of Joe Wilder, MD,* called "extraordinary" by *Sports Illustrated. Art News* recently published a featured profile on Dr. Wilder, and his works have appeared in numerous major galleries and in private collections. He describes himself as a visceral rather than a cerebral artist: "When I paint Ali fighting Frazier, I *become* Ali. It is my juice, my energy, my anger, my strength transmitted to Ali's fist through my paintbrush."

As Virginia Woolf well knew, a Beethoven quartet really is the truth about the world. As she might have guessed, given life enough and time, an electron micrograph is also the truth about the world. So is Edward Hopper. And Mozart. And Einstein and Roentgen and Faulkner. And Constable, who went so far as to say that Art is a Science. All windows open to the same world.

When those windows open to the arcane and intricate blue-green world of the surgeon, no pair of artist-scientist-surgeons could be better equipped for an aesthetic collaboration than Seymour Schwartz and Joe Wilder. For these two have given their lives and talents to surgery, to the human encounter which is medicine, and to Art with a capital *A*. In this book the art of each marries very well the art of the other. To appropriate from the language of molecular biology, their aesthetic "receptor sites," each for the other's work, are a most felicitous, often revelatory, fit.

When I think of surgery, I think of Emily Dickinson's quatrain of advice to its practitioners:

Surgeons must be very careful
When they take the knife!
Underneath their fine incisions
Stirs the Culprit—Life!

Drs. Schwartz and Wilder, each in his own inimitable, wide-ranging, and provocative fashion, are just as careful when they take up pen or paintbrush. And we are all richer for the care, the love, with which they do so—richer because, so often, these two artists have framed and captured for us "an eternal moment" from out of this ever-various world.

Allow me one more quote that seems especially appropriate for the artistic collaboration at hand. It's from John Ciardi, the late poet, translator, and wordsmith, from his poem "The Gift." The poem concerns one Joseph Stein, a poet and a survivor of Dachau, and one of the lessons he learns, not only about writing, but about *all* art. The lines remind me always of just how triumphant, sustaining, and renewing the work of the artist can be, as this book so eloquently attests:

Clean white paper waiting under a pen
Is the gift beyond history and hurt and heaven.

John Stone, MD

I have known Sy Schwartz and Joe Wilder for a long time as surgeons and humanists, but I never expected that they would invite me to make introductory comments. Each is an esteemed producer in the "art book" genre, so in retrospect I should not have been surprised by their collaboration; both are broad-gauge overachievers in several fields.

Overachievement connotes for me preeminence in a major field of endeavor, plus outstanding productivity in other areas often far removed from one's primary profession. Dr. Schwartz is a well-known cartophile; not merely a lover of ancient maps but a respected expert and author in the field. He is also an eminent editor of surgical texts and journals and a department chairman distinguished for his research, teaching, and administration. I have long admired his executive participation in leading national and international organizations.

Dr. Wilder's phenomenal talents and tenacity were evidenced early by his unparalleled achievements in lacrosse at Dartmouth and by his skilled success in caring for the seriously injured Zero Mostel, who in his gratitude introduced Joe to individuals at the cutting edge of modern art, such as Jasper Johns. The ordinary aspiring painter seeks guidance by lessons, but for Joe the autodidact method was more congenial. By his own description, he flung himself into painting and frenetically flung paint at endless canvases, until his early daubs gave way to dynamic paintings of sports figures, surgical scenes infused by a deep personal intuition, and still lifes of a captivating intensity.

Both cartography and surgery comprise science and art. There are major technical aspects to graphic arts, aside from the personal inspiration, the artistic conceptualization, and the historical antecedents that convey aspects one might wish to imitate or avoid. Surgeons and other professionals such as painters are a part of the political milieu; in this they function as change agents through their work and their philosophy.

The scientific leverage of space exploration has brought to cartography both new vision and undreamed-of precision. In art the provenance of old masters has been revolutionized, at times disturbingly, by new radiographic imaging. And medical essayists have been challenged in their ethical fundamentals by technical advances.

It is stimulating and inspiring to read the evolving succession of the Schwartz editorial comments selected from a quarter-century of perceptive analysis. These are juxtaposed against relevant paintings by Joe Wilder, another surgeon whose art has matured pari passu with his own philosophical evolution and with that of his partner in this unique collaboration. Here are variegated gems to be savored and treasured.

C. Rollins Hanlon, MD, FACS

Foreword

Images in Paint...

Throughout my career as a teacher and a Chief of Surgery I have taught that the operating room should be seen as a cathedral in which all occupants should respect the sanctity of this space. All attention should be focused on the patient and the mission to be accomplished—namely, successful surgery. I never permitted loud talking or jokes or stock market discussions, and I continue to believe that a quiet ambience should be pervasive, with the same respect and quiet that we show in our places of worship.

I have tried in my surgical paintings to portray the surgeon as the dedicated, caring, hard-working individual I have observed by the thousands in my 35-year career as a Chief and Professor of Surgery. Still, my surgeon series is but an extension of the joys I have experienced and the many things I have learned these past 35 years while painting all manner of subjects: athletes, racing cars, landscapes, seascapes, and with deep joy, the sweetness of still lifes.

Joe Wilder

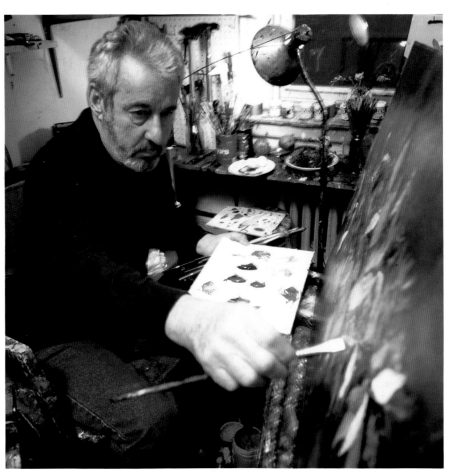

Claude Etinger and *ArtNews*

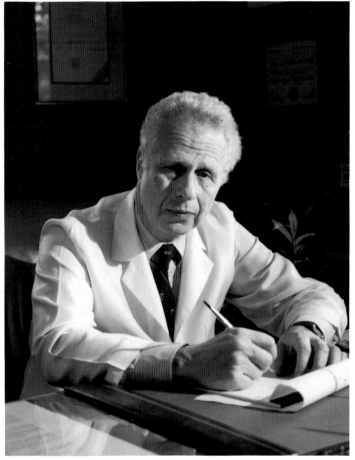

David Bruce

...And in Prose

The artistry of surgery requires a mastery of science, an assimilation of experience, and a perfection of technical skills for the proper assessment and management of a clinical problem. But because that clinical problem is only one focused element of a complex human being, surgeons must relate to patients holistically. In constant dialogue with patients concerning issues of suffering, life, and death, the surgeon benefits from an appreciation of literature and art, images of the past and present.

The complete surgeon not only acts but thinks, not only thinks but feels. The surgeon cries and laughs, worships heroes, deposes devils, dreams and reflects, and creates personal images.

We two practicing surgeons have expressed our images in two different media, using words and colors, for over two decades. Here we have coapted our efforts within this binding for the pleasure of our medical colleagues and all the people we care for.

Seymour I. Schwartz

Preface

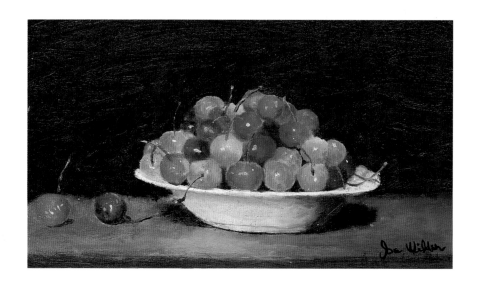

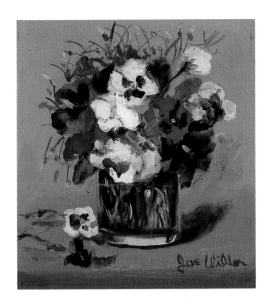

PART FIVE

Ethics and Education

PART SIX

Obiter Dicta

PART SEVEN

Communication

Contents

Contemplation Before Surgery. It is here, at this moment, in the midst of the quiet bustle of the operating arena, that the surgeon stands finally alone, hands clasped in the classic aseptic position, in a loneliness only he can know. In this last moment before action, he stands in contemplation, in a prayer of supplication. It is now that he draws from the past, that he brings to bear all his knowledge, skill, and expertise in the service of another person. Working with the known, he enters the unknown, whose final outcome can be known only when it is no longer possible to change it.

M. Therese Southgate, MD, Cover Editor, Journal of the American Medical Association

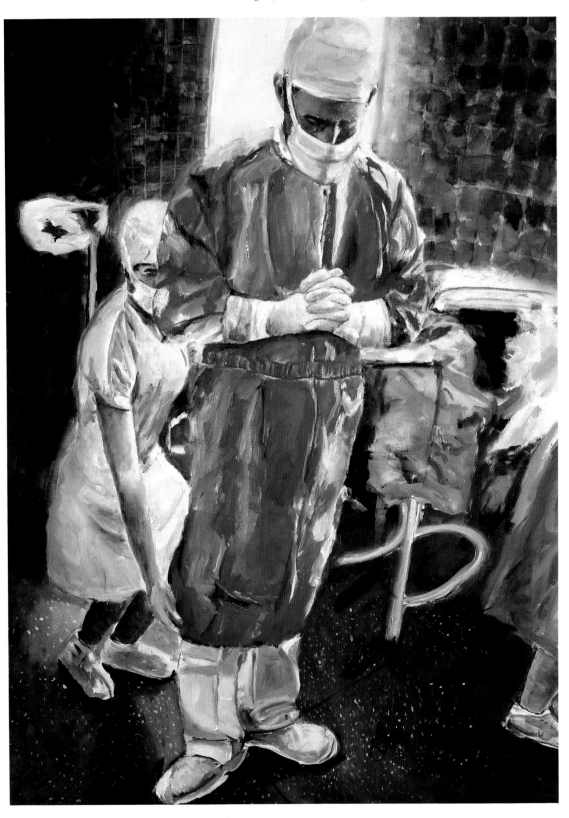

*T*hroughout the second half of the twentieth century we have lived our medical lives in an explosive era of excitement. The achievements that are currently commonplace would have been unanticipated and unrecognizable by the generations that immediately preceded us. Entirely new fields of cardiovascular surgery and transplantation have developed and rapidly expanded. It has been an age of technical advances with computer tomography, ultrasonography, magnetic resonance imaging, and fiberoptically improved endoscopy to facilitate diagnosis. Staples and scopes have been produced to expedite surgical management. We have begun to use monoclonal antibodies and genetic and immunologic manipulations and we have corrected anomalies with intrauterine operations.

Surgery and medicine have been transformed; when we look to the future we anticipate that transformation will continue as the dominant theme and that it will occur at an accelerated pace. There will be extraordinary technologic refinements in the realms of instrumentation and automation. Refined and expanded immunologic modulation and genetic manipulation will rapidly become commonplace clinical applications. New words, new formulas, new concepts, and new therapeutic algorithms will evolve. Today's information explosion will be magnified to inconceivable dimensions. Tomorrow's computers will facilitate the processing of this information, but the human brain will remain a limiting terminal.

As we focused on scientific facts and logical conclusions, our cells for cerebration accommodated to a wealth of knowledge. Our synaptic processes have effected sequences that have expeditiously resolved theoretic and practical problems. As a consequence, as physicians and surgeons, we have extended life at both ends. More premature babies live and an older population survives critical illnesses and major interventions. We have developed new cures and have fashioned more elaborate repairs and reconstructions. As physicians and surgeons, we have succeeded and will continue to succeed in addressing and resolving our patients' physical ailments and disorders.

In this scientific scenario, has the third law of Newtonian physics applied? Has there been an opposite and equal action? Has the gain been offset by a loss? Has the humane element that was emblematic of our profession waned? As we have provided more sophisticated care, has there been less caring?

An affirmative answer to these questions led to the current concern, which in turn created an impetus for the introduction of humanism into the curriculum of medical schools and as part of continuing medical education. "Humanism" is the devotion to human interests; it has no distinct formulas, no absolute numbers, no data. Humanism

Reflections

may be temporal, at times ethereal, but nevertheless the devotion to human interests is a real factor. It may pertain to given situations or to small segments of a single situation. Humanism, although disparate from our usual data orientation, provides a powerful and meaningful force that should influence our clinical attitude.

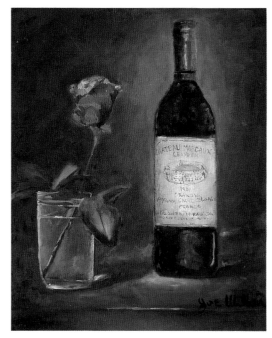

Based on our scientific and technocratic conditioning, humanism is often inadvertently relegated to a minor role in our performance. Classic liberal education has given way to focused education. Focused education throughout the physician's continuum of learning has consumed the limited time for learning and has created an impersonal mind-set responsive to specific data. The resultant combination of required focus and constraint of time impedes or precludes the acquisition and assimilation of that corpus of learning known as the humanities.

In ancient Greece the term "humanities" referred to "a polite scholarship such as grammar, rhetoric, poetry, and classics." In modern times it generally incorporates philosophy, literature, and the arts concerned with human culture.

By absorption of the thoughtful expressions and analyses of diverse literary works, by the emotional impact of prose and poetry, by the sensate response to an oil painting or a concerto, by the humbling effects of an appreciation of history and its heroes—all a part of humanities—humanism will evolve. The gains from reading literature, viewing art, and listening to great works of music are personal and professional.

On the personal level, in a time that such a concentrated and major energy is required to remain current in the science of medicine, the humanities fulfill the need for an important intellectual addendum. They generate emotional gratification by

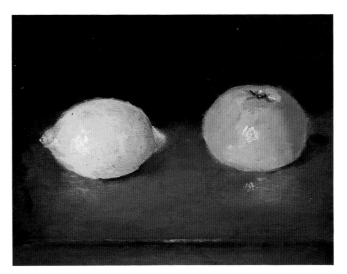

providing the condiments to make more palatable a constant diet of surgical and medical science. Appreciation of the past that led to the present state of the art of medicine, exposure to the thoughts of the leaders in previous generations, and recognition of the heroic proportions of the activities of those who have preceded us add romance to rote. Learning becomes more pleasurable. The arts can only amplify the science of medicine. It is appropriate that

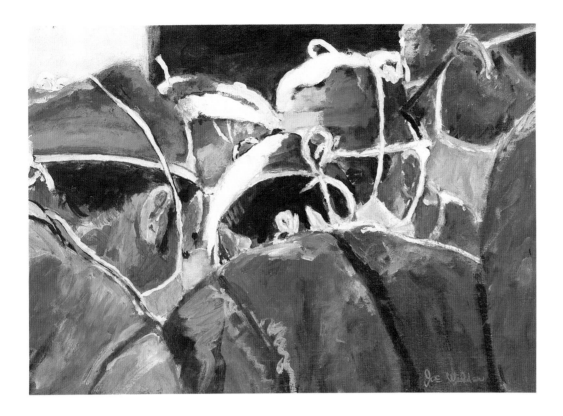

St. Luke is not only the patron saint of medicine but he has also been designated the patron saint of artists.

The impact of the humanities on professional performance is potentially equal if not more significant. The practice of medicine and surgery with its expanded scientific base will forever remain part art because the patient is an individual and as such has unique responses to the same stimulus. The unique psychologic and personal factors that impact on a given patient must enter into the physician's equation for management. Sympathy and empathy play a necessary role and they are incorporated in, if not the essence of, humanism.

We have written and painted in the hopes that the audience will read and regard, but more important, join in our reflections and our feelings. In the segments of our lives, exemplified by the contents of this synthesis of our two types of expression within one binding, we offer a token of participation in a curriculum in which humanities is emphasized. We have lived our lives as surgeons; we have taught the science of surgery and surgical techniques. This conjoined work is a presentation of a shared credo that more than science and technique must be taught and must be learned.

The study of the humanities makes the scientific individual more complete and more satisfied. Personal equanimity results. Prose and pain excite a feeling; feeling adds "caring for" to the "care of" patients. To the Cartesian dictum, *Cogito, ergo sum* (I think, therefore I am), a most meaningful extension is added, and we and our patients both benefit. As individuals we each loudly exclaim, *Cogito et sentio, ergo melior sum* (I think and I feel, therefore I am—better).

Seymour Schwartz

Miscellanea

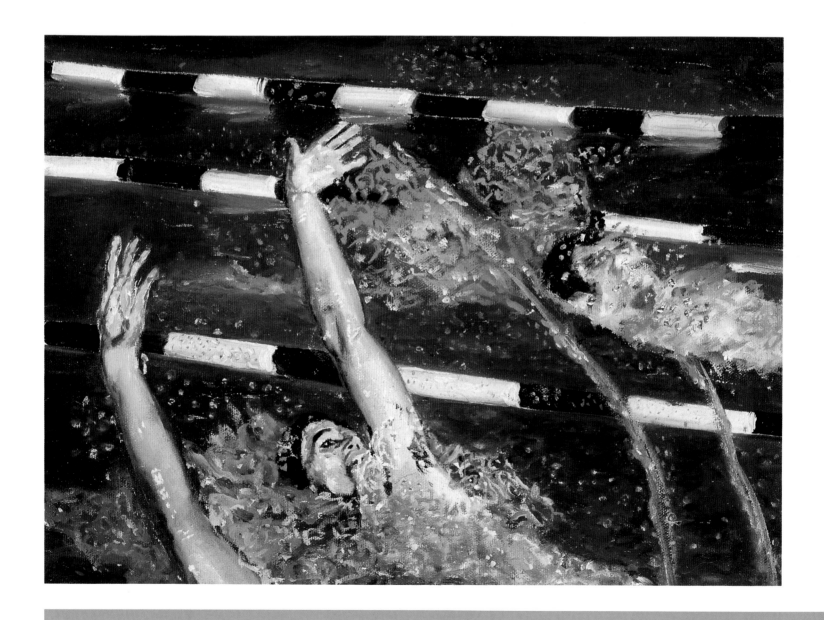

I celebrate the great contrasts in nature by painting athletes and animals performing extraordinary feats with their bodies as they leap, jump, race, sail through space—miracles of movement and living machinery; I derive equal joy from painting still lifes. It requires great discipline to capture the sweet fuzz of a peach or a watermelon seed or a tiny sap-green leaf, the opposites of movement—miracles of nature quietly reminding us there is harmony.

I am a visceral painter, not a cerebral painter. I am not interested in reproducing the botanical quality of a cherry or a leaf. I am interested in getting underneath the skin of the fruit and flower, making them come to life with a universal truth. My interest as a painter with the human form started as a young athlete, continued as a surgeon, and finally found permanent expression as an artist.

When I paint Nolan Ryan pitching, I *become* Nolan Ryan, and into that pitch goes my lifetime as a competitive athlete. As Ryan rears back to pitch, he is for that instant Joe Wilder throwing all of his life energies into Ryan's pitch. When I paint Ali fighting Frazier, I *become* Ali. It is my juice, my energy, my anger, my strength transmitted to Ali's fist through my paintbrush."

Long fulfilled and rewarded as a Professor of Surgery and Hall of Fame athlete, still nothing has given me the sheer ongoing joy of being a painter. Painting is all about using your eyes and seeing better the world around you. William Carlos Williams, the physician and poet, said it best and I join him, "I like most my ability to be drunk with a sudden realization of seeing things others never notice." And it is all for free.

Throughout my career as an athlete, surgeon, and painter, I have struggled long and hard with society's obsession with stereotyping us and squeezing us into a small slot. Painting has been the pathway to a long odyssey to being my own person and doing my own thing. I took Joseph Campbell's advice long ago: "If you are fortunate in discovering your bliss, take hold and never let go."

Finally, I look upon the world around me as my free province. This has to be one of the great joys of creativity, for creativity need not have boundaries and parameters. All of nature, all objects, all creatures great and small are mine for the painting—free—to be painted when and how and what and where it suits me. Humans and animals, still lifes, flowers, fruits, landscapes, seascapes, men and women and physicians and surgeons. They all beg to be painted, and if I am fortunate, I shall paint them all.

Joe Wilder

An Artist's Credo

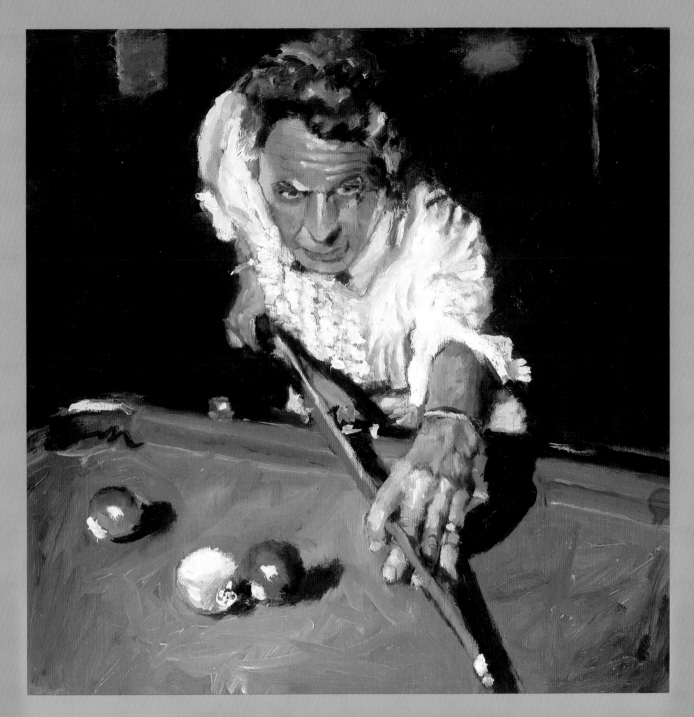

PART ONE

Culling From
the Calendar

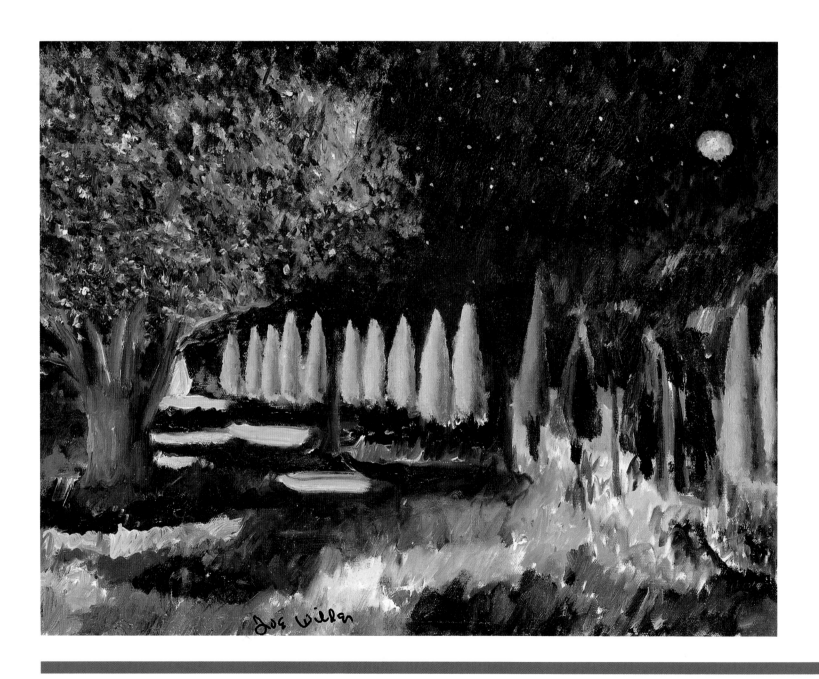

Moonlight Landscape. 1980. Oil on canvas, 14 x 18″.

The calendar, a remarkable achievement, is an expression of time that Daniel J. Boorstin described as man's first grand discovery in his highly recommended book, *The Discoverers*. By marking off days, weeks, months, and years, mankind liberated itself from the cyclical monotony of nature. Like many of our apparently immutable fact sheets, our present yardstick of time is a product of change.

The Babylonians developed a calendar based on the cycle of the moon. The Jews and Muslims persist in their adherence to a lunar calendar; Christianity maintains its ties to the lunar calendar, best exemplified by Easter, which is prescribed in the *English Book of Common Prayer* as the "first Sunday after the full moon which happens upon or next after the twenty-first day of March, and if the full moon happens upon a Sunday, Easter Day is the Sunday thereafter."

In the ancient Alban calendar in which the year had 10 months, April occurred first and consisted of 36 days. The month's name derives from "Aperio: I open," probably referring to the opening of flowers, symbolic of rebirth. In the Romulus calendar, April was the second month and had 30 days. Numa's 12-month calendar assigned April its present fourth place with 29 days, and so it remained until the 46 B.C. reformation of Julius Caesar, when it returned to 30 days. The Julian calendar, which contained 365 days and a Leap Year every fourth year, erred by 11 minutes and 14 seconds in its measurement of the solar year. Therefore, Pope Gregory ordained in 1582 that October 4 be followed by October 15 so that the equinox would occur on March 21 of the following year. To prevent future discrepancies, the Gregorian calendar omitted the leap day from years ending in hundreds unless they were divisible by 400. This is our present calendar.

The word "calendar" was derived appropriately from the Latin terminology for an accounts-due document. Residing on a wall, situated for closeup viewing on a desk, or folded within a binding to permit it to accompany us throughout the day, these gridded leaves of paper function as a reminder of our contracts with the future, our obligations at present, and our activities in the past. Appointments with our patients, scheduled operations, meetings, and ever-looming deadlines fill the dated spaces of our lives.

A Checkerboard for Living

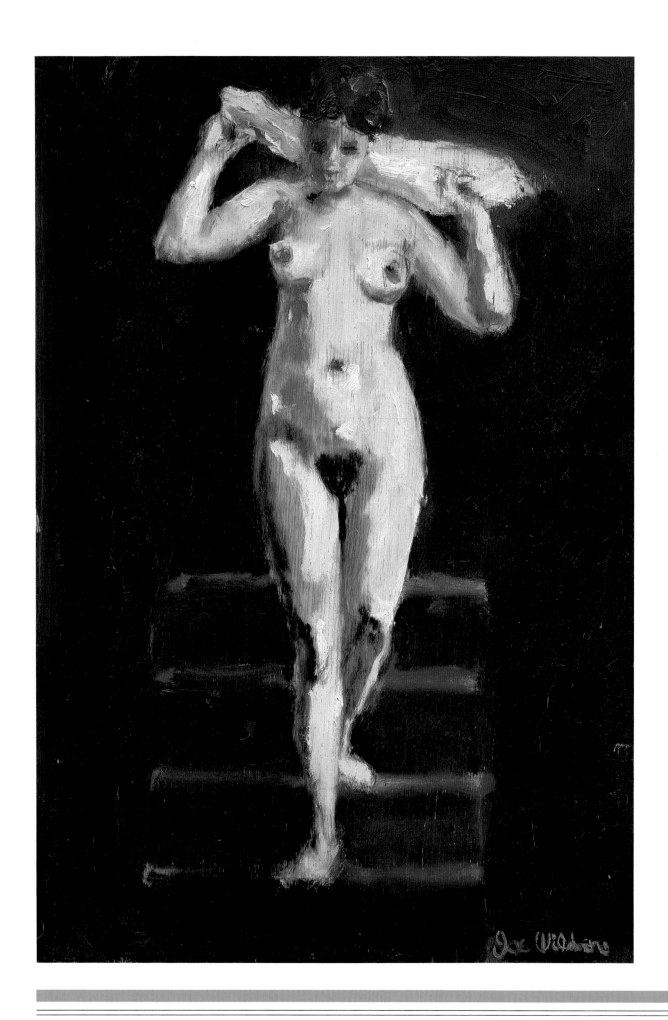

Nude Descending a Staircase. 1986. Oil on panel, 12 x 18″.

The year 1991 arrived and brought with it a relative rarity for a year, that is, a numeric palindrome—a number that is the same backward and forward. The most familiar verbal palindrome is Adam's alleged greeting to Eve: "Madam, I'm Adam." Palindromic famous names include Unu, the Premier of Burma, Laval, the Quisling Premier of France, and Lon Nol, of Cambodia.

But to return to palindromic years during this millennium, let's review them to define our progress. In 1001, Avicenna was the dominant medical authority. The University of Paris was founded about 1111 and Padua about 1221. In the field of trauma, firearms were first mentioned in 1331. The printing press that revolutionized education and communication was invented about 1441. The year 1551 saw the establishment of anatomic theaters at Paris and Montpellier. In 1661, Stensen described the parotid duct and Malpighi published the first account of the capillary system. In 1771, George Armstrong described pyloric stenosis and the Reverend Richard Price published the first actuarial table. It was during the previous year that the first medical degree in the United States was conferred, on Robert Tucker, at King's College in New York City.

In 1881, Billroth successfully resected the pylorus for cancer and performed a gastroduodenostomy. Wolfler introduced gastroenterostomy. Weiss, in Billroth's clinic, described postoperative tetany. New York Polyclinic was established as the first postgraduate American Medical School. The first Russian surgical (Pirogoff) society was organized.

The year 1881 also witnessed a historic event in American surgery: the first scientific meeting of the American Surgical Association. On September 13, 1881, at the improbable location of the Brighton Hotel on Coney Island, with Samuel D. Gross presiding over 11 members in attendance, only three papers were presented. Samuel W. Gross, son of the president and himself a professor at Jefferson Medical College of Philadelphia, reported on "The Influence of Operations Upon the Prolongation of Life and Permanent Recovery in Carcinoma of the Breast." R.A. Kinloch, professor of surgery at the Medical College of South Carolina at Charleston, presented a "Report of a Case of Supposed Spontaneous Aneurysm of the Posterior Tibial Artery," and a series of case reports was offered by John H. Packard of Philadelphia.

Returning to the written word, we can consider Napoleon's palindrome, "Able was I ere I saw Elba," and Ronald Reagan's assessment of Manuel Noriega, "A man, a plan, a canal, Panama," or the more easily structured line palindromes, such as "Bores are people that say that people are bores." If the subject is resurrected in the year 2002, "So patient a doctor to doctor a patient so," will still pertain.

Periodic Palindromes

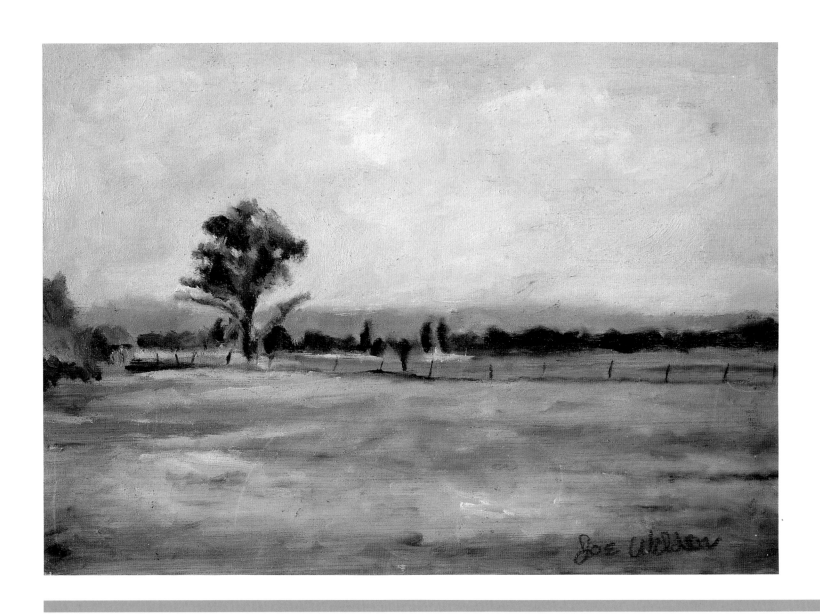

Pastoral Landscape. 1985. Oil on panel, 8 x 11½".

As we approach the twenty-first century and look back at our beginnings as American surgeons, it is appropriate to consider colonial times. None of the colleges in the Colonies had a medical department before 1760. Of the 3000 to 4000 individuals practicing medicine in 1776, no more than 400 had received medical degrees, mainly from the University of Edinburgh. The medical department of the College of Philadelphia was established in 1765 and the medical department of King's College, New York, in 1768. Only 51 degrees were conferred by these schools before 1776. The curriculum at the Medical College of Philadelphia pointedly excluded surgery, because "a physician should not be engaged in that discipline." Harvard Medical School was the third to be established, opening in 1783. Its authority to certify graduates qualified to practice medicine was immediately challenged by the Massachusetts Medical Society. The Society claimed that the legislature had granted it the right to examine and license candidates for the practice of medicine and surgery. Completing the roster of eighteenth century medical schools was the medical department of Dartmouth, founded in 1797, with Nathan Smith as its one-man faculty. The medical school of Transylvania University in Lexington, Kentucky, was founded in 1799 but did not open until 1817.

The only permanent public general hospital established during the colonial period was the Pennsylvania Hospital, opened in 1751. The New York Hospital obtained a Royal Charter in 1771 but did not function during the colonial period. The annual expense of the hospital was about $2000 to $3000, and the major criticism was that the hospital refused to accept sick patients if they had no money. The New Orleans Charity Hospital actually antedates New York Hospital as an operating institution, but New Orleans did not become part of United States Territory until 1803.

American medical literature was sparse before the Revolutionary War and included one medical book, three reprints, and 20 pamphlets. The book was written by John Jones, the first professor of surgery at King's College, and appeared in 1775. It was a compilation of several works of various European surgeons and contained only a single original observation. Only one medical journal, "Medical Repository," a quarterly edited in New York, existed in the eighteenth century.

Medical practice was consumed with the treatment of infectious diseases and the management of great epidemics of yellow fever and cholera. The precepts and teachings of Benjamin Rush dominated much of American medical practice. Rush believed that the disease was caused by accumulation of bodily poison that exerted its effect by causing

Colonial Times

a nervous constriction of the small blood vessels. His therapy was directed at ridding the body of poison and bringing about relaxation of nervous excitement. This was effected by inducing vomiting, purging, sweating, and bleeding patients.

Although extraordinary fees for services were received by English physicians and those on the Continent, in America the fees were most modest, even when rendered to exceptional people. George Washington paid approximately $38.50 for care of his family and 200 slaves. Before the Revolutionary War he paid a physician a fixed annual income of approximately $20 to render these same services.

Washington might have led the country along the road of prepaid programs and HMOs, but I wonder how he, and more appropriately, James Madison, the architect of the Constitution, would react to the current level of government control and bureaucracy. I further wonder whether, in an atmosphere of frequently ephemeral acronymic governmental agencies, a document like the Constitution could have been written by only 55 men in less than 4 months.

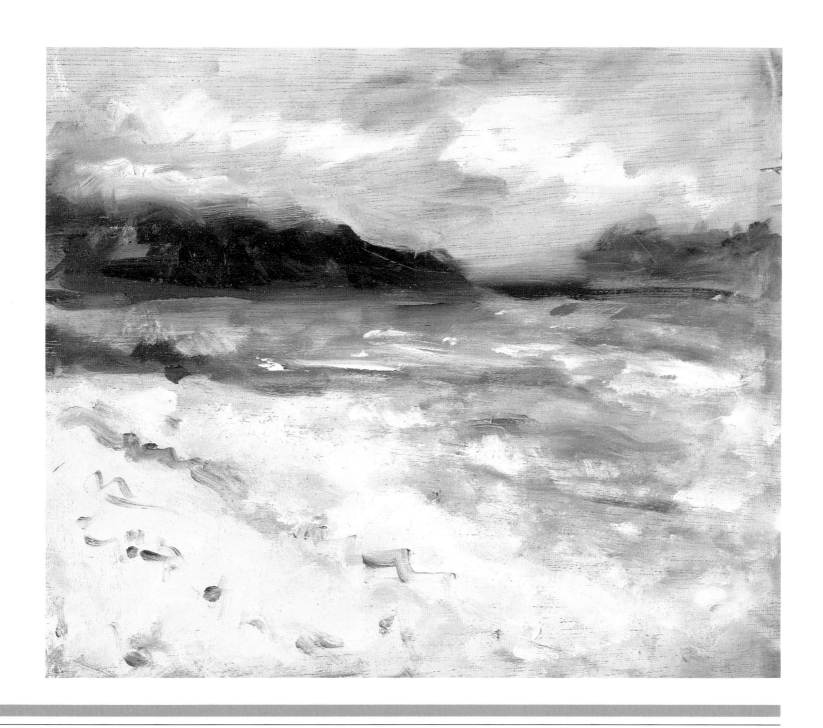

9 *Twilight Seascape*. 1992. Oil on panel, 8 x 9½″.

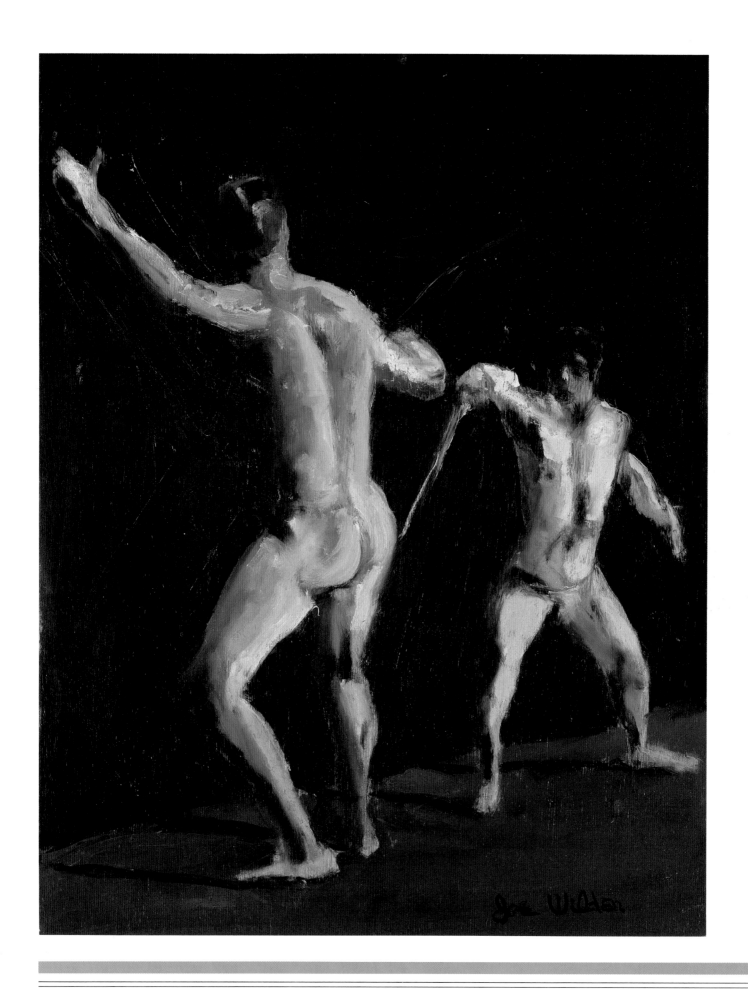

Fencers, after Muybridge. 1986. Oil on panel, 14 x 11″. Collection Margo Karlin.

The god Janus, for whom the first month is named, was endowed with two heads; one looked at the past and one at the future. Janus was also revered as the deity of doors. The characteristics attributed to Janus can be convoluted into an editorial reflection.

We have partially emerged from the prejudices and doctrinaire attitudes of the past. In our own lifetimes, there have been quantum leaps in surgical science and massive changes in the socioeconomic aspects of the practice of surgery. Most have been advantageous. As W.W. Babcock stated in the preface of his *Textbook of Surgery* (1928), "We shall not scorn what was done yesterday because we have something better today any more than our interest in the past will cause us to continue the practice of the past." We should pay homage to our heritage and honor our heroic surgical progenitors, yet heed the dictum of William Stewart Halsted in "The Training of the Surgeon": "It is now as it was then and as it may ever be; conceptions from the past blind us to facts which almost slap us in the face."

In 1948, Isidor S. Ravdin rightly predicted, "In the surgery of the future the individualist will be left by the roadside," as the field broadens and becomes more refined. This certainly has positive and negative implications, as we regard an intellectual milieu that emphasizes quantification and increased precision rather than initiation of broad concepts and as we strive in a socioeconomic atmosphere dominated by bureaucratic growth control.

But the worst of all possible personal attitudes would be one of passive pessimism. The words of Sir William Osler are appropriate: "Everywhere the old order changes, and happy are they who change with it." Individuality can be persistent throughout change. Herbert Spencer expressed an opinion that evolution was a change to coherent heterogeneity.

The past and future meet in an evanescent present, and we are temporarily enclosed in our confines. One door must be opened and closed to let in the positive parts of the past and to keep out the counterproductive elements. Another door must be opened to provide access to the avenues of the future, and at the same time closed to prevent movement along improper paths. The vision of temporarily residing in a room with swinging doors leads me to paraphrase a sentiment expressed in *The Rubaiyat of Omar Khayam:*

As I think of the past and places I've been
I've oft come out by the door I went in.

Janus:
A Two-Headed God

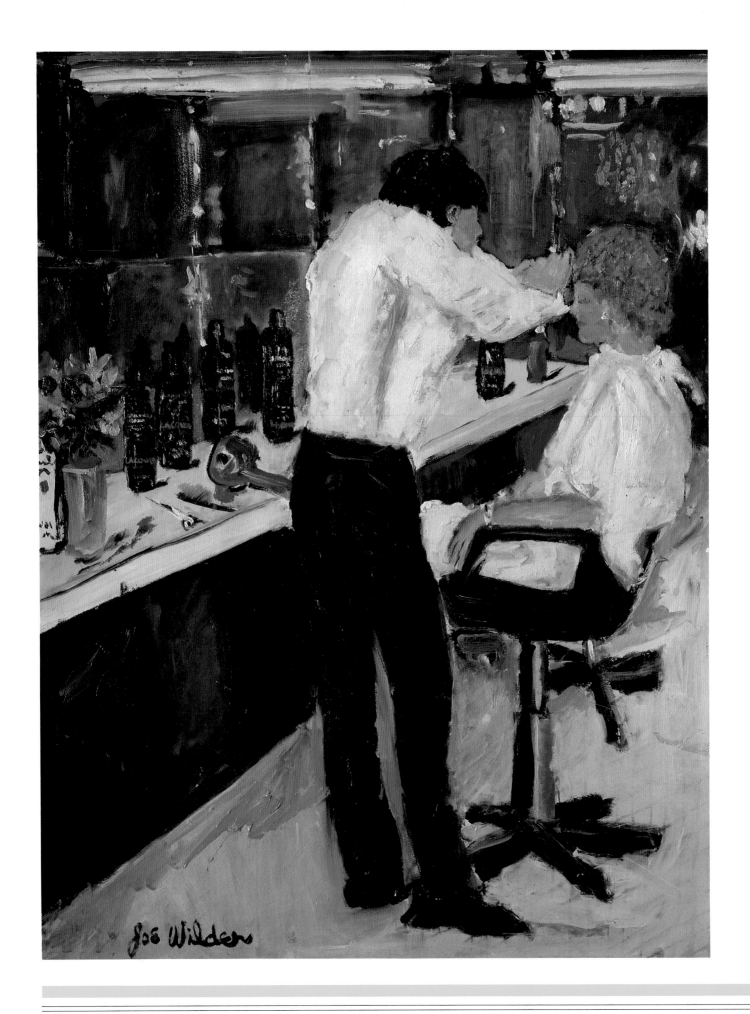

The Barber. 1990. Oil on panel, 24 x 18″.

The lion that "roars in the beginning of March" brings to mind another lion, closely related to our surgical heritage. That lion occupies a central position on the cross of St. George that is part of the arms of the Company of Barber-Surgeons granted by Queen Elizabeth I in 1569.

The association between barbers and surgeons began in 1123 when a papal decree ruled that a priest who shed blood was debarred from higher office. The Barbers' Gild probably began in the thirteenth century, but the earliest direct reference to the Gild is in the naming of its first known Master, Richard le Barber, in 1308. Between that time and 1540 there were two separate organizations concerned with the practice of surgery in London: the "Company of Barbers" and the "Fellowship of Surgeons." As an increasing number of members in the Company of Barbers became engaged in the practice of surgery, they took on the title "Barber-Surgeons Company." In 1369, three master surgeons were sworn in to supervise the practice of surgery in London. In 1462, King Edward IV granted the Barbers' Company its Royal Charter.

The Gild, or Fellowship of Surgeons, was a smaller, more select organization that also existed in the fourteenth century. In 1493, an agreement was reached between the two groups, and, as a consequence, two wardens were appointed from each side to regulate the practice of surgery in the city. During the same period, changes were occurring throughout the continent. On March 7, 1515, in Padua, Italy, the fight for recognition of Barber-Surgeons was achieved when, for the first time, a university degree of Doctor of Surgery was conferred on a surgeon who had no knowledge of Latin.

The union of the Barber-Surgeons Company of London and the Fellowship of Surgeons is regarded as one of the most important events in the history of surgery in England. The act of Parliament received Royal Assent on July 25, 1540, and this was considered so significant that the organization commissioned the great Holbein the Younger to paint a picture of Henry VIII presenting the Charter. Our current barber pole is actually a representation of the early days of the English barber-surgeon. The white stripes symbolize the bandage, the red is for blood, and the gilt knob commemorates the brass basin used to catch the blood.

There is evidence that toward the end of the seventeenth century the surgeons were discontent over their union with the barbers, and in 1745, by an act of Parliament

Tonsorial Times

and Royal Assent, the barbers and surgeons were separated. That year, the Royal College of Surgeons held its first meeting. On March 22, 1800, the Royal College of Surgeons of London was established by a Charter from George III.

The most literary of the Barber-Surgeons was perhaps William Clowes (1540-1604), who marched to the same drummer as those of us who have compiled textbooks. In 1591, he published *A proved Practice for all young Chirurgians*. His second book, *A profitable and necessarie Booke of observations,* included his poetic consideration of a surgical cure:

> Hippocrates in his aphorisme, as Galen writeth sure,
> Saith, foure things are needfull to every kinde of cure.
> The first, saith he, to God belongeth the chiefest part,
> The second to the Surgeon, who doth apply the art.
> The third unto the medicine, that is dame Natures friend,
> The fourth unto the patient, with whom I heere will end.
> How then may a Surgeon appoint a time, a day or houre?
> When three parts of the cure are quite without his power.

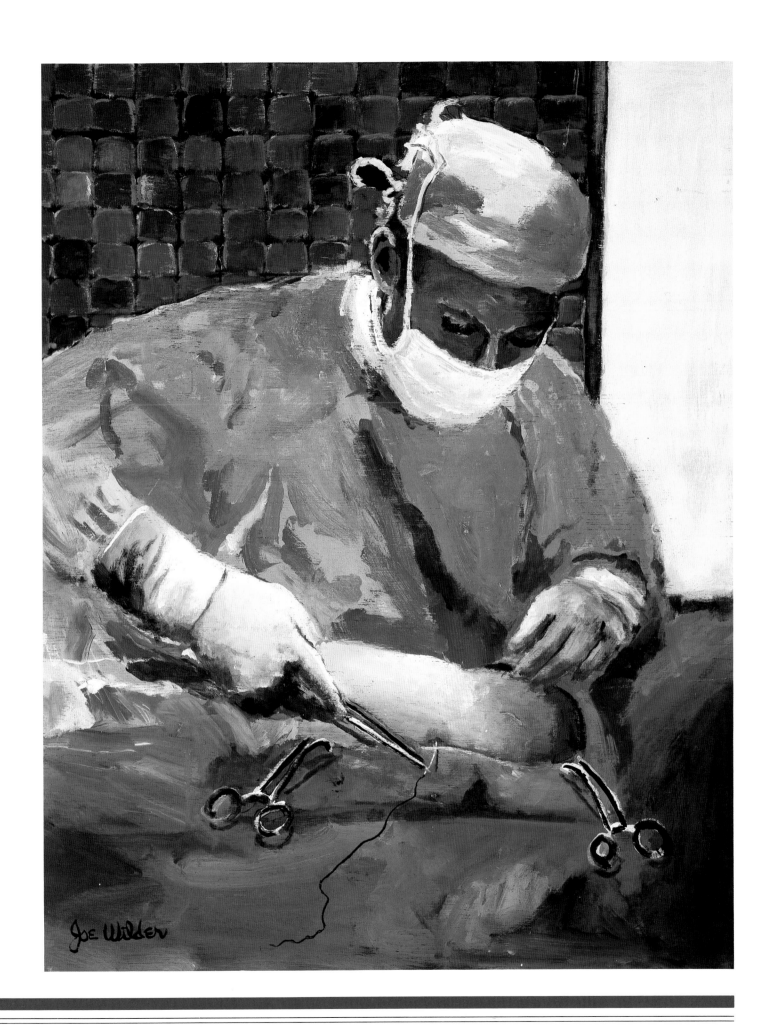

15   *The Surgeon.* 1989. Oil on panel, 24 x 20″.

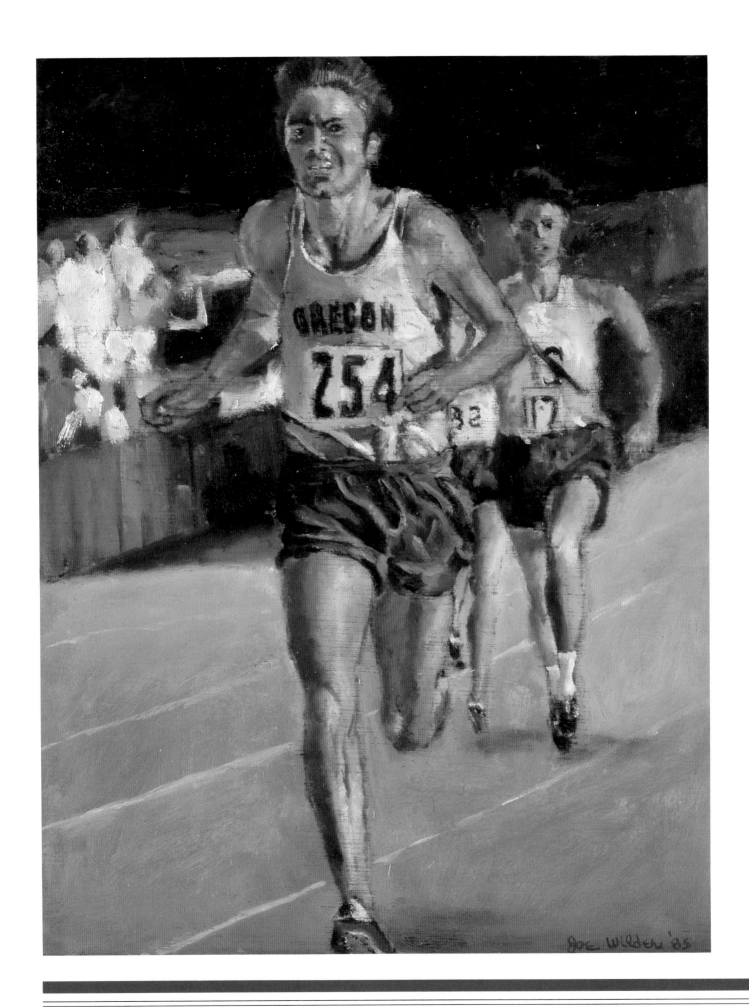

Prefontaine Breaking the Record. 1985. Oil on panel, 12 x 12″.

In Poor Robin's Almanack for 1760, it is written, "The first of April some do say, is set apart for All Fools' Day, but why the people call it so, nor I nor themselves do know." A day that the ancient Romans consecrated to fools brings into focus several aphorisms and notable considerations.

Antedating the refinements of vascular surgery, George Ross stated in the latter half of the nineteenth century, "Any fool can cut off a leg—it takes a surgeon to save one." In a sense of bravado, Sir Heneage Ogilvie published in Lancet (2:1, 1948) a restructuring of the famous Oslerian statement, "A surgeon who is his own physician, though he often has a fool for a colleague, has the happiness of working in an atmosphere of mutual confidence and admiration."

On a more serious note, it is important constantly to remind ourselves that every major discovery in science represents a criticism of things as they are, and therefore, the wise man generally evolves from one who had been considered a fool. Charles Darwin said, "I love fools' experiments." And John Homans, a major force in American surgery, is quoted as saying, "I prefer to be called a fool for asking the question rather than remain in ignorance."

It was on April Fools' Day in 1578 that William Harvey, the greatest of the discoverers in the field of physiology, was born, and it was during three days in April 1616 that he delivered the first statements of his thoughts on the circulation of blood. With creditable reserve, 12 years elapsed before he published the most famous of all of his works, *Exercitatio Anatomica de Motu Cordis et Sanguinis in Animalibus*. In his great work, Harvey wrote, "What remains to be said upon the quantity and source of the blood which thus passes, is of so novel and unheard-of a character that I not only fear injury to myself from the envy I feel, but I tremble lest I have mankind at large for my enemies, so much doth wont in custom, that become as a second nature, and doctrine one sown and that hath struck deeproot, and respect for antiquity influence all men."

Thus, in April, the opening day of which is dedicated to the fool, let us honor one who was born on All Fools' Day, and pay homage to the fact that from the ranks of those we presently regard as fools come those we are eventually willing to follow in reverence.

Fools Become Leaders and Wise Men Followers

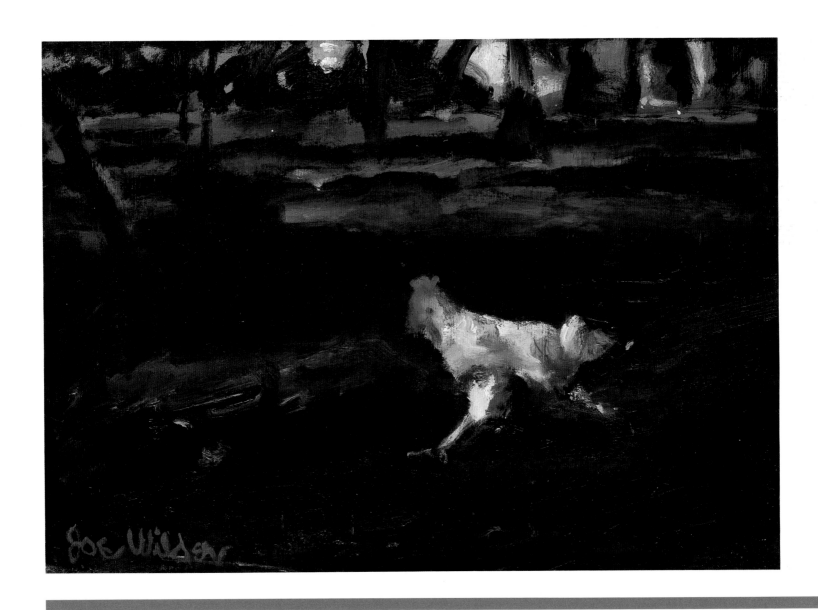

Gauguin's Rooster. 1985. Oil on canvas, 8 x 11″. Collection Cynthia Wilder.

The month of May has been designated National Humor Month, and it is timely to reaffirm the tripartite importance of humor and laughter in our surgical behavior. Humor can play a critical role in the patient's process of coping with the stress of illness. Similarly, humor can mollify the emotional trauma of surgical training and can actually serve as a catalyst in the teaching-learning dialogue. Finally, we need to laugh at ourselves as an integral part in the development of our personalities. Humor, humility, and humanism all appropriately begin with the same three letters.

For the diseased patient, humor bolsters morale, contributes to a sense of well-being, and has been credited with having a biological survival value. Pindar wrote in the fifth century, "The best of healers is good cheer." Nietzsche was more forceful when he declared that "Man alone suffers so excruciatingly in the world that he was compelled to invent laughter."

For the students and residents we are privileged to teach, humor can stand out as an important ingredient in the educational process. Humor was defined by Stephen Leacock as the "kindly contemplation of incongruities of life." Humor has been identified as a means of facilitating learning, and as Ralph Waldo Emerson pointed out, "We must learn by laughter as well as by tears and terror."

Perhaps the most important target for humor is ourselves. Emerson's quotation was preceded by the sentence, "The perception of the comic is a tie of sympathy with other men, a pledge of sanity." The title of the English periodical devoted to humor, *Punch*, probably was suggested from the name of a medieval Italian comic figure Punchinello, which in turn came from the Italian word "polcino," meaning chicken or rooster. We all possess an element of comedy as we strut through life, even though we deal in serious matters. It is not necessary to be so imbued with the gravity of our charge that we totally subjugate imperfections and the laughable facets of our personas. Laughing at one's self is a manifestation of strength and not weakness. We can be reassured by Thomas Carlyle, who said, "No man who has once heartily and wholly laughed can be altogether irredeemably bad."

Humor, Humility, and Humanism

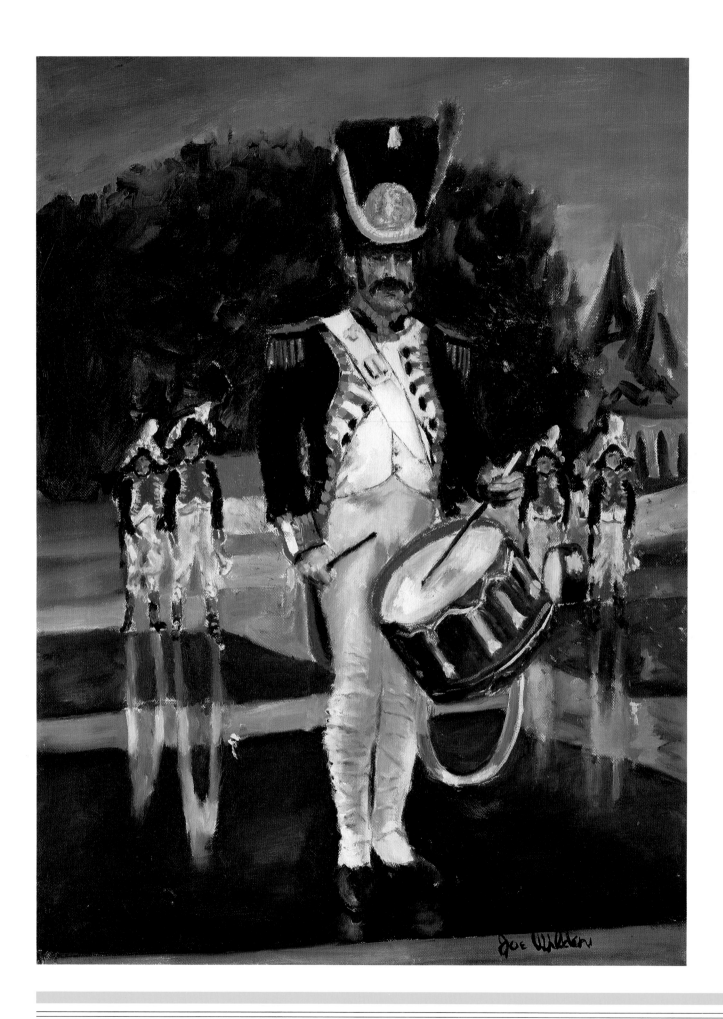

French Band, Statue of Liberty Celebration, July 4. 1986. Oil on canvas, 16 x 12".

*J*uly is ushered in with fireworks celebrating the Declaration of Independence for our country. John Adams said, "The second day of July, 1776, will be the most memorable epoch in the history of America." It was on that date that the resolution was passed proclaiming that the United Colonies ought to be free and independent states. On the fourth day of the month the document was approved and signed, making the United States the first country with a precise birthdate.

The beginning of the month of July also witnesses another declaration of independence when the surgical resident completes a training period and undergoes an overnight metamorphosis to become an independent surgeon bearing ultimate responsibility. As George Santayana wrote, "Declaration of Independence makes nobody really independent."

Although the essence of the practice of surgery, with its ever-increasing complexity, necessitates interdependence with others who bring varied expertise, this should not negate the Oslerian aphorism that "the most precious of all possessions is mental independence." It is essential that individual independence be allowed to exist and to flourish in an ambience of interdependence. This is certainly true when the investigative process is involved. Cardinal Newman addressed this issue in *Christianity and Scientific Investigation*, stating, "The investigator should be free, independent, unshackled in his movement."

The concept of independence is also nuclear to the clinical practice of surgery; it mandates that the individual have a consecration that is entirely from within. We all know that independence provides opportunity for transgressions, but the risks of the abuses are less worrisome than the consequence of nonindependence. Among the *Sayings of Napoleon* is the declaration that "Independence, like honor, is a rocky island without a beach." The intrinsic beauty of the island far outweighs the inconvenience of stubbing one's bare feet on a pebbled beach.

It is appropriate at this time to consider the "Ode to Independence" written by eighteenth century physician/author Tobias Smollett:

Thy spirit independence, let me share!
Lord of the lion-heart and eagle eye,
Thy steps I follow with my bosom bare,
Nor heed the storm that howls along the sky.

Pyrotechnical Pensiveness

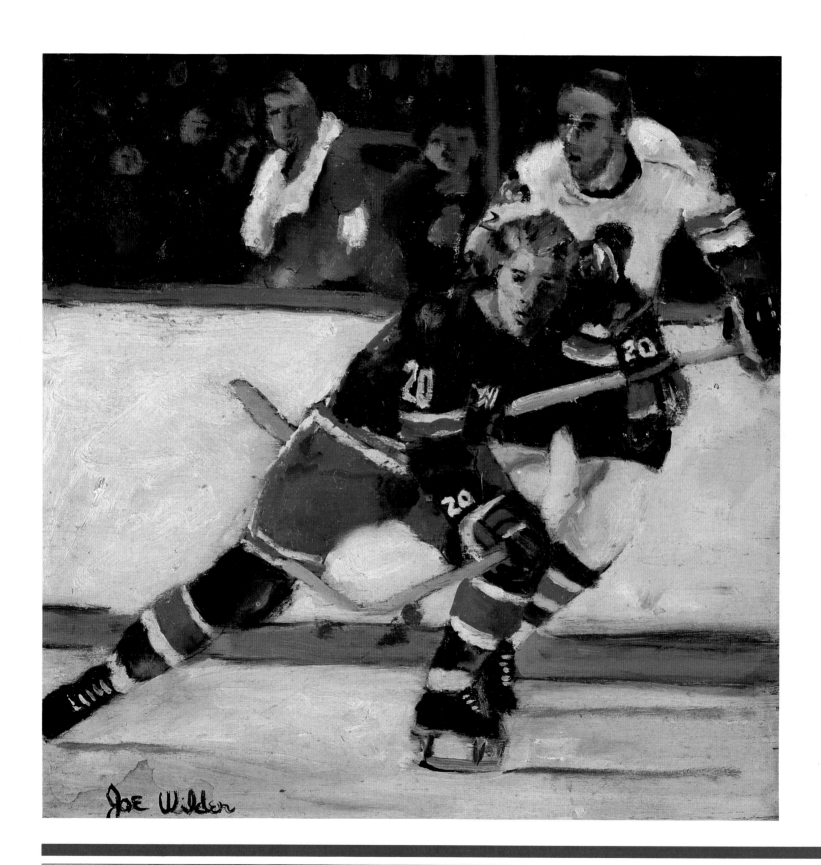

Hockey Playoff. 1991. Oil on panel, 12 x 12″.

I recently attended a medical school graduation ceremony at which I could not recognize the name of the keynote speaker. As he stood at the lectern, sporting hair that hung to the interscapular level and issuing statements about love for patients, generalities regarding medical care, and reciting a poem by T.S. Eliot, I remarked to the spectator seated next to me, "He's either in family medicine or pediatrics." My identification was correct.

One night many years ago while skating at an indoor rink, a surgeon, who was enjoying an evening of recreation, became a participant in the management of a sudden cardiac arrest in a fellow skater. The surgeon immediately took charge and called upon a medical confrere present to initiate mouth-to-mouth ventilation while the surgeon applied external cardiac massage. Among the skaters was an ophthalmologist, who volunteered to assess the extent of pupilary dilation. The group of physicians participating in the care of an emergency event became a quartet when a psychiatrist, who had also been skating, indicated that he would control the shocked crowd of onlookers and attempt to address their psychologic trauma.

These vignettes lend support to the thesis that, in general, there are relatively distinct personality traits characteristic of physicians practicing specific specialties. The surgeon remains unique in response to crises by early decision and action. This is doubtless the result of an individual's basic personality that contributes to the selection of a career, coupled with years of training and subtle influences by the personalities of surgical mentors and members of the peer group. Both the mentors and peers contribute to the amplification of a surgeon's appreciation of the signals of crisis and the speed of the synaptic process by which the surgeon acts rapidly when addressing a life-threatening medical problem. Appreciation of the precious factor of time, so often neglected by the nonsurgeon intrigued by the dilemma of diagnosis and the multiple technologic tools to affirm and reaffirm clinical conclusions, is an integral part of the surgical personality.

These editorial considerations are timely if you permit the circuitous routes of personal reflections. It is November. The month that saw the birth of Ephraim McDowell on November 11, 1771 and the first great operating gynecologist, J. Marion Sims, on November 13, 1813 could be regarded as a surgical domain. November is the eleventh month of our calendar; it was the ninth month in the old Roman calendar. It was derived from the Latin "novem," meaning ninth. Amalgamating nine and eleven resulted in the number 911, the universal emergency phone code, to which the surgical personality is particularly responsive. The surgeon should be regarded as November's child.

November's Child

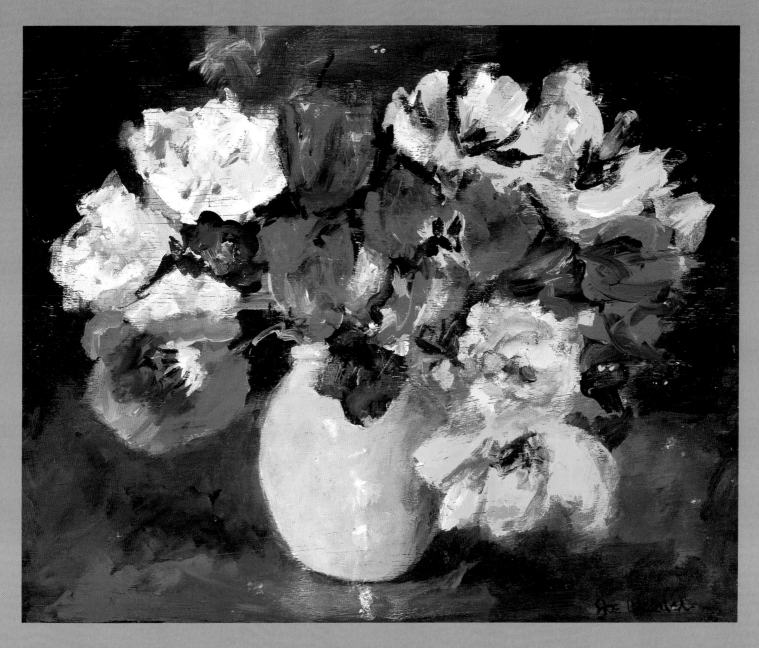

PART TWO

Changes

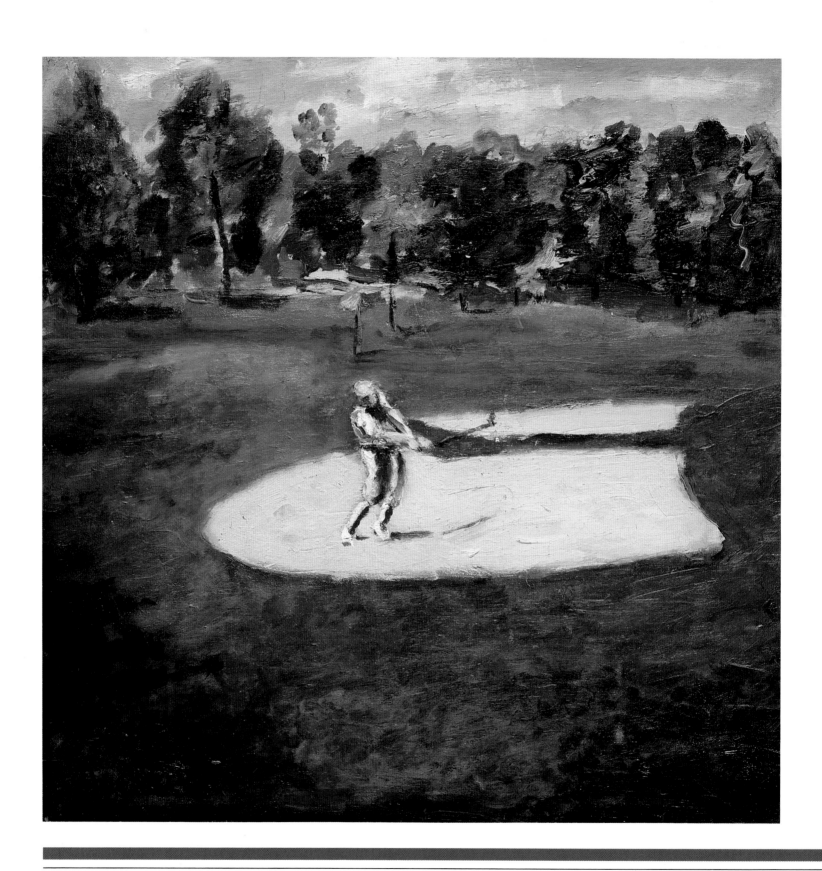

Out of the Trap. 1989. Oil on panel, 12 x 12″.

Two years ago my assessment of laparoscopic cholecystectomy was that it would not have the wide application that it has today. I made a major misevaluation and miscalculation. Thomas Huxley wrote, in *Science and Education,* "Next to being right in this world, the best of all things is to be clearly and definitely wrong. If you go buzzing between right and wrong, vibrating and fluctuating, you come out nowhere; but if you are absolutely and thoroughly and persistently wrong, you must, some of these days, have the extreme good fortune of knocking your head against a fact that sets you all straight again."

I am certainly willing to join any Greek chorus of recantation about the applicability of laparoscopic cholecystectomy. But I hope that surgeons do not evolve into laparoscopic zealots whose efforts are doubled when they lose sight of their goals. Mesmerization by novelty and technology is dangerous. The scenario of a recent novel might come to pass: the ventriloquist becomes enslaved by his inanimate dummy.

The scopic vistas have expanded within all the body's cavities. The list of lesions and organs removed and structures repaired is rapidly becoming more encompassing and approaches that of conventional operations. Through the scope, diagnoses have been established. Solid viscera have been "morcellized" and extirpated through ports, the dimensions of which are but a small fraction of the organs' size. Anastomoses have been fashioned with elegant miniaturized stapling devices; scope-guided suturing and tying techniques have been perfected.

Since the operative procedures are performed based on a two-dimensional image on a screen, binocular vision for depth perception is no longer required. The sensation of touch can also be dispensed with. Even one-eyed lepers are no longer impeded. The recent generation that has devoted significant time and effort to honing skills in Nintendo computer-generated games has fortuitously been preparing itself for adeptness as technical surgeons. Lewis Carroll would have been amused to note that an amalgamation of the titles of two of his most famous works, *Adventures in Wonderland* and *Through the Looking Glass,* anticipated the future of surgery.

To Err Is Human and Even Sublime

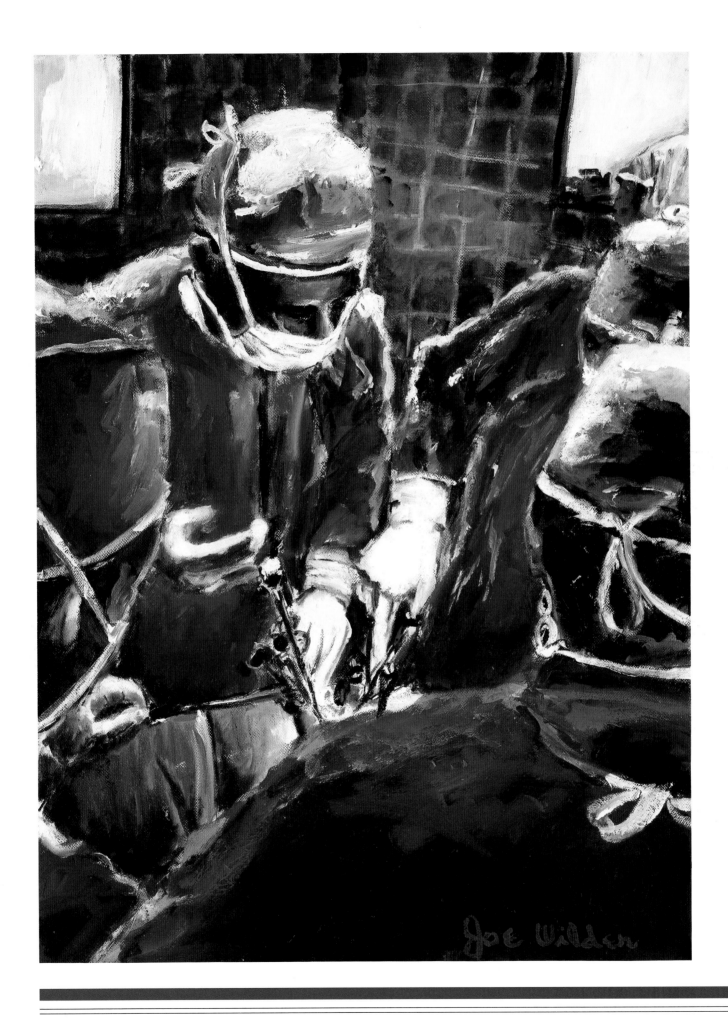

Operating Team. 1987. Oil on canvas, 16 x 12″.

The name Johns Hopkins instantly evokes thoughts about the modern concept of surgical training. The contributions of Drs. Halsted and Blalock have had major evolutionary if not revolutionary effects. Dr. Halsted's disciples have also had their time of influence. One has only to scan the list of Dr. Blalock's residents to appreciate the extent to which one institution has generated leadership in surgery. Drs. Halsted and Blalock are dead, and the circumstances on which their concepts of surgical training were predicated no longer pertain. The idea of using wards of indigent patients for the nurturing and maturation of surgeons in training has become unacceptable to our society.

Today, essentially all patients are categorized as "private," if the dominant financial yardstick is used. The current training of surgeons must be reconciled with this private patient population. Privacy defies precise definition. Implicit is the right to be left alone, encompassing the concept of autonomy.

In an age of litigation and consent forms, the therapeutic contract between physician and patient must be given greater consideration. It should be appreciated that if these two are to become partners contractually, the public must be educated to a level of understanding. The diffusion of medical culture among the nonmedical public becomes a social priority in achieving ethical therapy.

As part of this consumer education, the public must be apprised of society's future need for surgeons and of its associated obligation. This can be accomplished only by stressing the team approach to therapy and by overtly basing the contract between physician and patient on "supervision" and "responsibility" rather than on "technicality." The same public that has engineered a society characterized by the belief that all patients are entitled to equivalent care cannot remain ambivalent about the use of these patients to educate surgeons for the future.

As de Tocqueville wrote in 1835, it can be anticipated that Americans will be receptive to this change: "[Americans] consider society as a body in the state of improvement, humanity as a changing scene, in which nothing is, or ought to be, permanent; therefore what appears to them today to be good may be superseded by something better tomorrow."

Another quote expressing care about the future is that of John Buchan (Lord Tweedsmuir), who, on the occasion of the coronation of George VI, stated, "We can only pay our debt to the past by putting the future in debt to ourselves." Finally, a more personal selling point was made by Charles F. Kettering: "We should all be concerned about the future because we will have to spend the rest of our lives there."

The Changing Scene

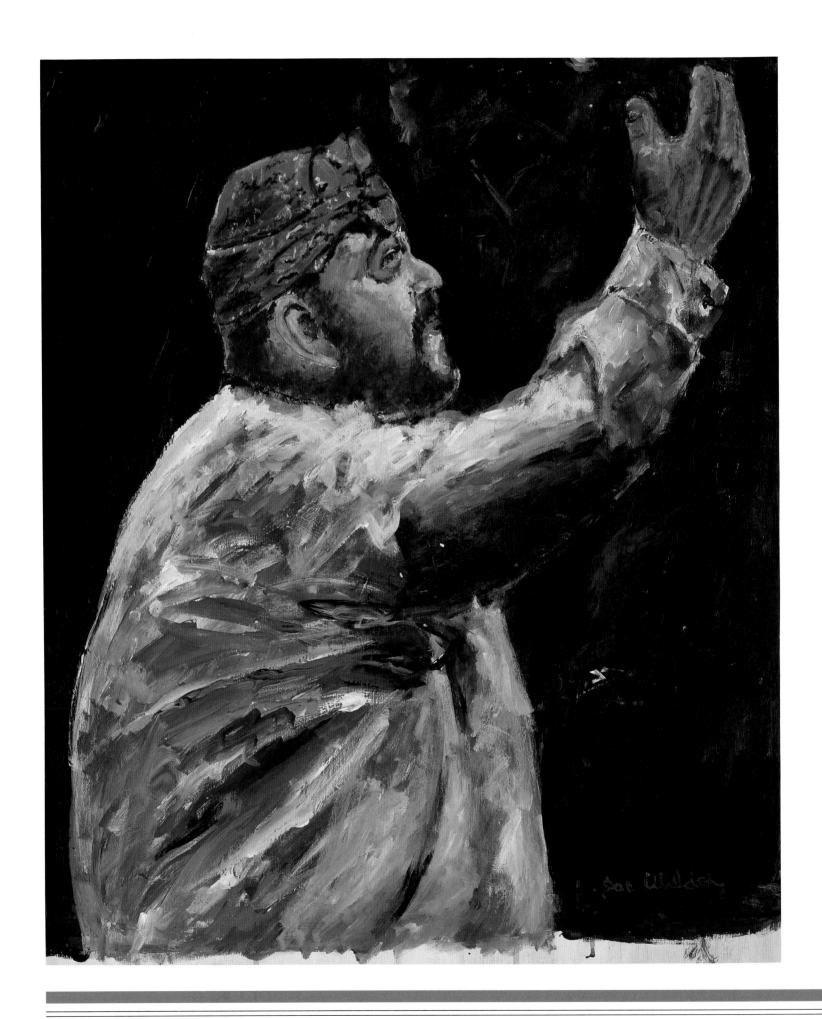

Zero Mostel. 1992. Oil and acrylic on panel, 28 x 24″.

The advent of the Professional Standards Review Organization (PSRO) is but one manifestation of change in the old one-to-one physician-patient relationship. The relationship is now a matter of public responsibility. The specter of regulatory organization is disturbing to many, because it is antithetical to *tradition*. The feelings of the concerned physician are not unlike those of Tevye in *Fiddler on the Roof,* confronted with a sequence of increasingly profound changes in his family relationships. The doctor's monologue might sound something like this.

"Why should I, an ethical, competent, concerned physician be harassed because a few of my colleagues don't meet the standards?

"On the other hand, I can hardly argue with the altruistic purposes of review—exclusion of malefactors, reward of excellence, and general improvement. Because of the experience with Medicare and Medicaid, a case was made for having adequate peer review to provide a mechanism for avoiding aberrant medical practice.

"On the other hand, the problems of review are (1) confusion about purpose and goals—is the focus on cost containment or quality of achievement? (2) confusion about the method of audit and quality of assessment, and (3) confusion about anticipated responses and extraprofessional pressures—will the program provide feedback and will it be predicated on a system of reward or punishment?

"On the other hand, quality care has long been a concern. In 1914, Codman advocated an accounting system to assess the quality of hospital care. The American College of Surgeons developed a program of hospital inspection, and in 1933, the Lee-Jones report addressed itself to the fundamentals of medical care.

"On the other hand, how widely will the results of a physician review be disseminated? Who will challenge whom? Examination of past experiences reveals the absence of a holistic approach and significant disarray."

The fiddler on the roof is loudly playing a new tune. It cannot be drowned out by shouting "Tradition!" We have two roads to choose from: One will move us toward increasing government regulation, the second toward a self-regulatory system that we ourselves build in the public interest. We cannot stay where we are, and, as the author of *Future Shock* reminds us, "Change is upon us: we resist it at our own peril."

A New Tradition

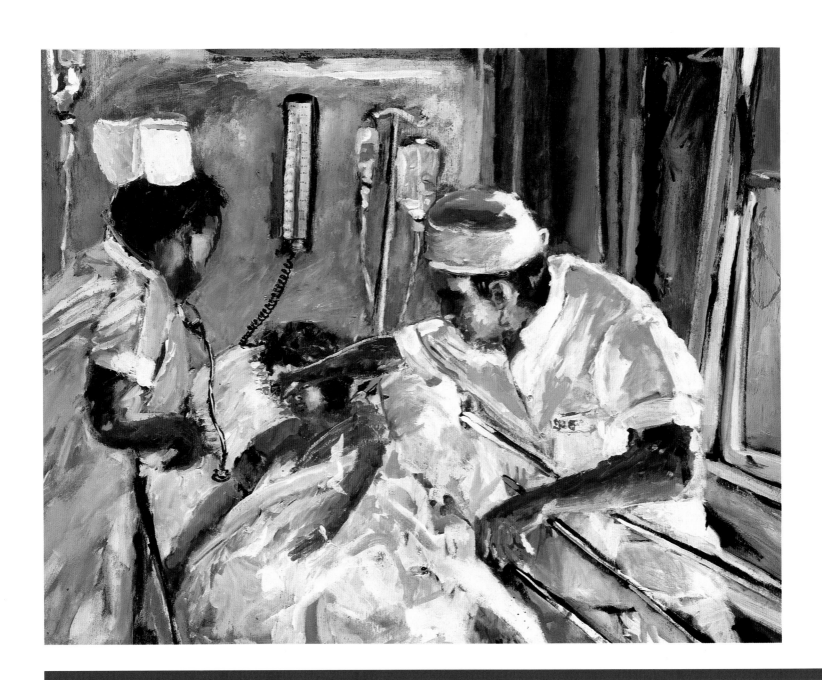

Recovery Room. 1990. Oil on panel, 22 x 28″.

*P*resently the pervasive and dominant conversations among all physicians, even the alleged Brahmins of Academia, relate to finances. The initials CC and DRG, designating Cost Containment and Diagnosis-Related Groups, could connote Concern over Control and Doom-Related Governance. One result of the plans for fiscal constraints could be applauded, however, because it will stem a potential flood of attitudinal change regarding the practice of surgery.

I recently learned that a leading academic orthopedic surgeon has said that orthopedic and perhaps all surgical patients should be admitted for work-up on the medical service and transferred to the orthopedic or surgical service via the operating room. I also heard the statement by the chairman of a Department of Medicine that responsibility for the surgical intensive care unit should be in the hands of the department of medicine because surgeons have neither the qualifications nor the time for that facet of care. The patients would be managed by a panel of experts, including nephrologists, cardiologists, infectious disease physicians, respiratory therapists, neurologists, and so on, all functioning with the cohesion of a symphony orchestra.

This scenario negates surgeons' responsibility for the totality of their patients' care—a perception that patients and the courts still hold. I do fear that in the jousting grounds of hospital administrative committees and academic councils, the surgeons would lose the battle because the numbers are stacked against them and there is no *amicus curiae*.

But an odd ally has appeared—economic concern that this approach will cost more! The death knell of these inappropriate incursions on surgical care may be rung not by the appreciation that these proposals regarding both admitting policies and intensive care can lead to the destruction of the patient-physician relationship, the neglect of total care, and the disappearance of humanistic role models for students and residents, but by the cash register. Just as the type of proposed surgical care has the potential of a *reductio ad absurdum,* so the cost could rise *ad infinitum.*

Four hundred years ago, in 1585, 108 settlers were left on the island of Roanoke off the Carolina coast to establish the first English settlement in the new world. Deliberately included were several specialists with varied expertise: a physician, a metalurgist, an artist, and a leading mathematical scientist. What resulted literarily was an elegant verbal and illustrative description of the geography, flora, and fauna. What happened literally was lack of direction, squabbles, famine, and rampant illness. The colony died.

Declining Dollars

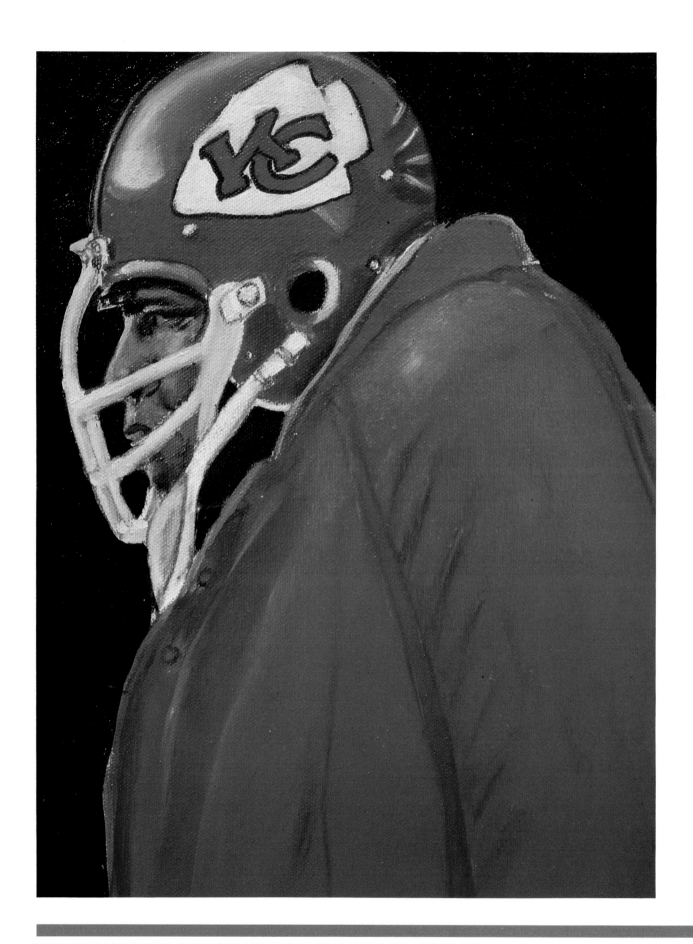

Buck Buchanan. 1975. Acrylic on canvas, 32 x 16″. Collection Dick Schaap.

Sports spectators will note that a frequent if not dominant chant at athletic events is "Defense! Defense!" With the evolution of specialty teams, as in football, many coaches feel the defensive unit contributes as much to victory as the offensive unit, if not more. Given the two approaches to the game, it is the team that defends successfully that wins.

Medical practice has also evolved so that now a defensive element tempers the physician's diagnostic and therapeutic approaches. This is the practitioner's attempt to guard against potential litigation. "Informed consent," originally intended to protect patients, has been emphasized, studied, and expanded to protect the providers of medical care.

It is extraordinary that so much centers on a document that implies physician-patient distrust. It is a return almost to the attitude held in ancient times, when therapeutic failure could spell loss of life, limb, or sight for the physician. Many points can be raised about the informed consent document and its refinement. I focus on only two—an ethical and an economic one.

First the ethical aspect. In the decision by the Supreme Court in the case of *Imbler v Pachtman* (No. 74-5435), it is stated that "the public trust of the prosecutor's office would suffer if he were constrained in making every decision by the consequences in terms of his own potential liability. . . . [It] would have been thought in the end better to leave unredressed the wrongs done by dishonest officers than to subject those who try to do their duty to the constant dread of retaliation." Can this reasoning not be extrapolated, in part, to other servants of society, that is, physicians and surgeons?

Second, the economic consideration. At a time when there is national clamor about escalating health care costs, the process of informed consent should be cost accounted. Ultimately, the patient or system underwrites the preparation and printing of the document as well as the time spent by the staff detailing and explaining the almost limitless potential physical and emotional effects of an operative procedure.

The informed consent document is merely a set of words intended to communicate understanding. As such, it can never be complete. Language can only approximate meaning. Furthermore, legal linguistics cannot successfully address the issue of "atmosphere." Energy and money spent refining such documents would be better applied to improving the environment in which physicians treat and patients are cared for. Defensive medicine, with its economic and emotional consequences, is a pollutant byproduct of society that should be eradicated.

Defensive Medicine

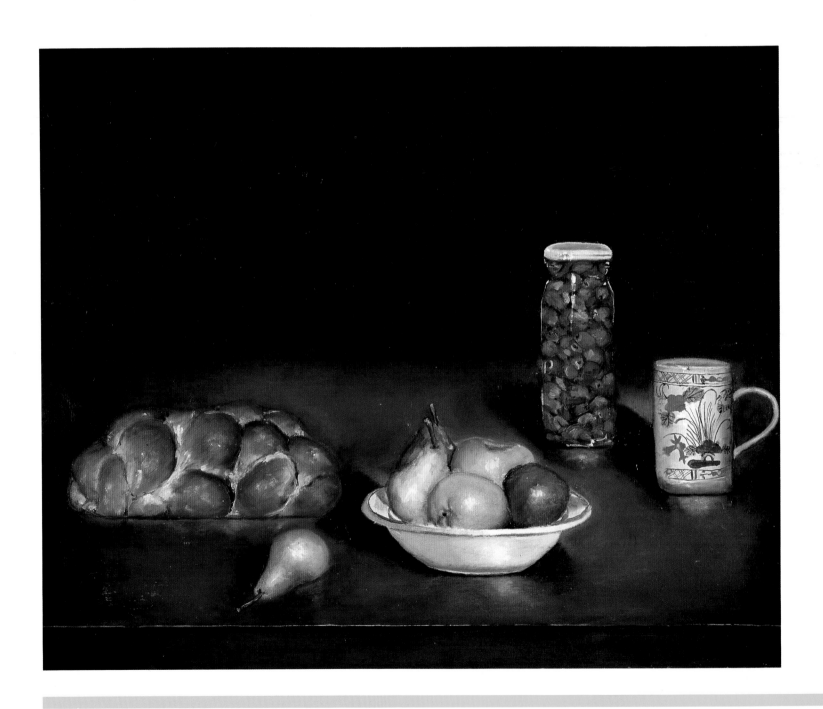

Still Life: Challah, Summer Fruit, Sentinal Pear. 1982. Oil on canvas, 24 x 30″.

The technical achievements of home dialysis and home-delivered total parenteral nutrition are in concert with a growing appreciation of the importance of the home environment for patient care.

As is the case with most hallowed institutions, the hospital has undergone a sociologic evolution. The hospital was considered a psychologic boon by Elizabeth Barrett Browning in *Aurora Leigh* when she wrote, "How many desolate creatures on earth have learnt the simple clues of fellowship and social comfort in a hospital." At the same time cries against the attitudes within hospitals were exemplified by the statement of John Fisher Murray in the *World of London*, 1850: "Tell her she can't be allowed to die in peace; it is against the rules of the hospital." In 1916 the distinguished surgeon, Charles Mayo, enunciated his strong feeling: "The sooner patients can be removed from the depressing influence of general hospital life, the more rapid their convalescence."

The hospice is proposed as a new popular concept for chronic care. The concept, in fact, is as old as the word, which according to the *Oxford English Dictionary* has the exact same derivation and original meaning as the word hospital—a house of rest and entertainment for pilgrims, travelers and strangers. For many, the home provides the optimal ambience for recovery from or coping with illness.

The modern hospital should be reserved for acute care, which cannot be achieved on an ambulatory basis. Early discharge of patients to their homes has obvious psychologic implications of comfort, security, familiarity, and reduced personal cost. The societal byproduct is the better use of institutional space.

Thus, as we regard our postoperative patients and reflect on their sluggish recovery and despondency, it is appropriate to bear in mind Witter Brynner's poem, "The Patient to the Doctors":

Name me no names for my disease
    With uninforming breath
I tell you I am none of these
    But homesick unto death.

Home Caring

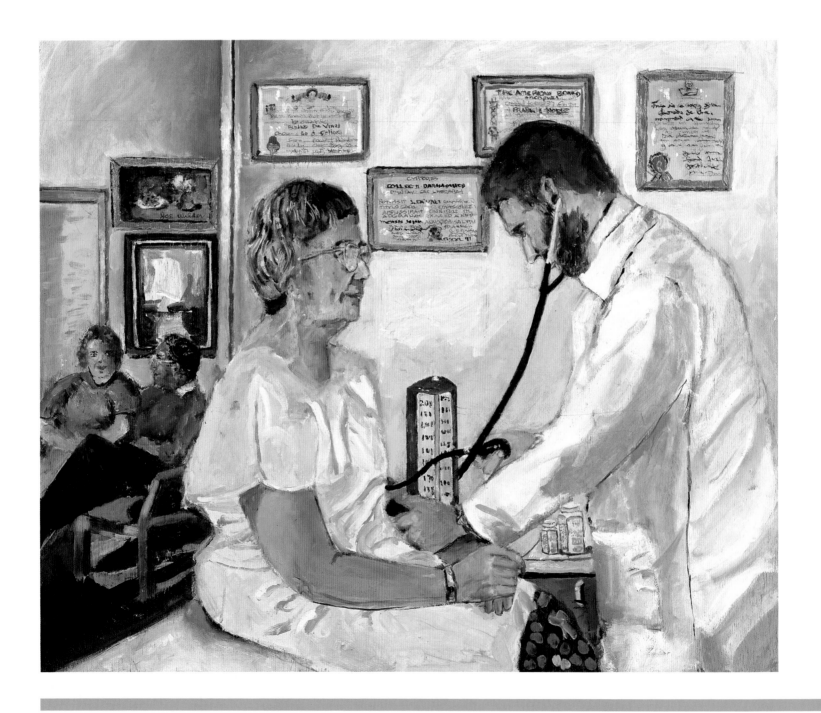

The Healer. 1991. Oil on canvas, 20 x 24″. Collection Pfizer Labs, a division of Pfizer Pharmaceuticals.

Refinements in biochemical techniques and the routine screening of multiple determinations at a practical, low cost have led to atrophy of the clinical intellect. Routine use, based on economic advantage, of screening panels negates the development of an important clinical attribute—the critical selection of appropriate diagnostic studies. Computer evaluation of the results of a battery of tests will further divorce the clinician's cerebration from the patient. The physician may come to be regarded as a "satellite station" that merely bounces information from a computer terminal to a patient terminal.

The explosion in diagnostic refinements has had a tremendously positive effect in the management of many diseases. But it is time to pay heed to the statement made by David Seegal in 1962: "One of the unexpected and disturbing results of the development of increasingly precise and useful diagnostic measures in the laboratory and x-ray departments is a significant and often alarming decrease in emphasis on the training of the medical student to perform with excellence the average comprehensive physical examination."

The role of the clinician, a word that literally means "at the bedside," has been altered. The venue of perioperative interest has changed, and the clinician has become further detached from the patient as a complex organism. There is no test that can define the patient's reaction to pain or detail the general nutritional status and other interrelated problems. Palpation of a pulse tells much more than the intensity of that pulse or the state of the circulation through the large vessels, because when the pulse is palpated it is evaluated by a physician in contact with a patient.

Perhaps we should stay the rush to transport the patient to the diagnostic noninvasive laboratory and recall the statement of Archimathaeus from about the twelfth century, "The finger should be kept on the pulse at least until the hundredth beat in order to judge of its kind and character."

Feeling

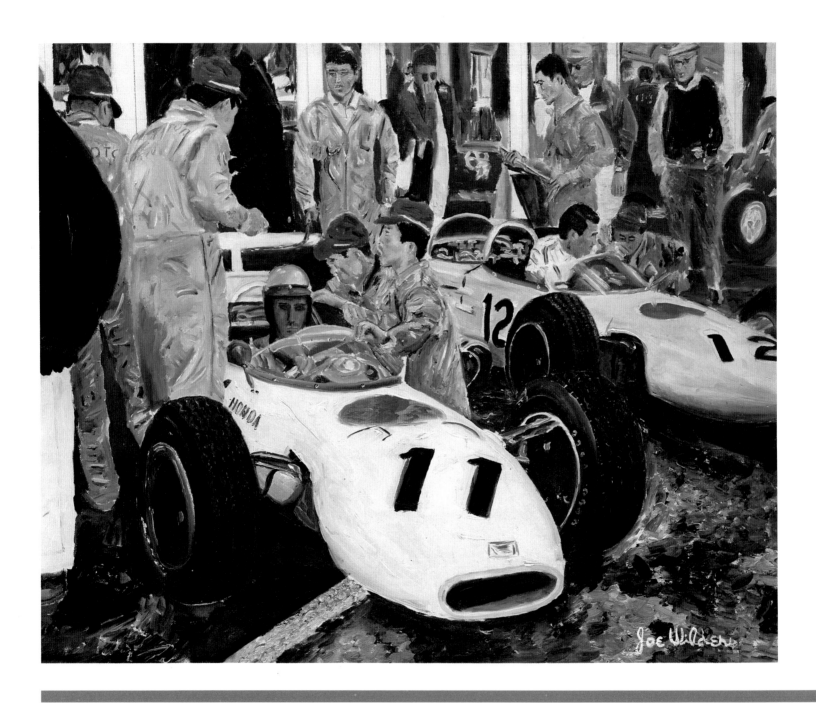

Grand Prix–Formula I–Honda Group. 1967. Oil on canvas, 30 x 24". Collection Cynthia Wilder.

*F*ifty years ago there were no computers. Now everyone has been or will be affected by these machines and their programs. Michael Crichton, the well-known author on this subject, has made several pertinent statements: "People are more important than computers. A computer is easy to use; this is fortunate because everyone is going to have to learn. It is not easy to use *wisely;* that is unfortunate because everyone is going to have to learn."

There is little doubt that in the realm of management of a physician's practice, retrieval, storage, and generation of medical information, the panoply of usages of numbers, the silicone chip and its serial circuitry will plan an integral role. We must become conversant with its applications but at the same time remain aware of its limitations.

Gilb's law of reliability states that "at the source of every error which is blamed on the computer are at least two human errors, including the error of blaming it on the computer." Before assigning superhuman unerring powers to the computer, it is essential to heed Peter Drucker's aphorism that the computer is basically a moron and the IBM Pollyanna Principle that machines should work and people should think. Just as an expert may be one who avoids small errors while sweeping on to a grand fallacy, so a computer may magnify a minor error into a total foul-up.

As we rely more on computer readouts, computer-generated diagnoses, physiologic profiles, and therapeutic algorithms, it is important that the machine remain the slave. In that regard, the combination of the patient's history and the physical examination should maintain its primacy. But even more important is the recognition that the computer will never be able to generate the sine qua non of medical practice—compassion.

Although I have become a devotee of the dedicated word processor and the home computer, I still echo the words from Hamlet's letter to Ophelia: "Oh dear Ophelia, I am ill at these numbers. I have not art to reckon my groans."

Bits and Bytes

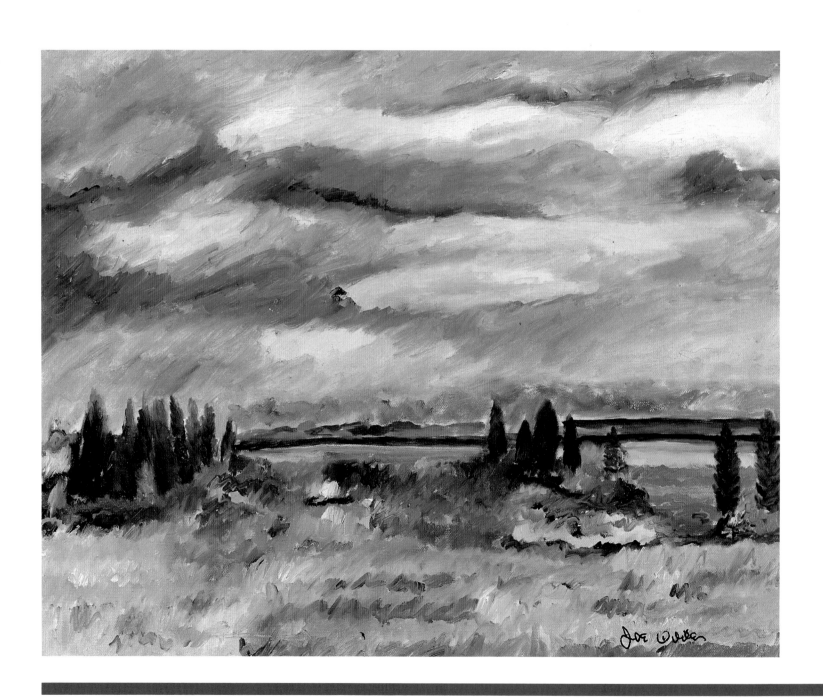

Stormy Spring Landscape. 1980. Oil on canvas, 16 x 20″.

A symposium during which therapy of a given disorder is discussed by representatives of different disciplines reflects the daily practice of medicine. In the past the surgeon generally indicated that the availability of excellent anesthesia and the support of sophisticated blood banks, coupled with improvement in instrumentation and the surgeon's own skills, permitted more liberal excision of offending pathology. On the other hand, the radiation therapist supported the ability to achieve cure with minimal side effects as a consequence of refined equipment. The chemotherapist suggested that the latest combination of old and newly introduced drugs constituted the preferred treatment, while the internist exclaimed that none of these measures had been demonstrated to be totally effective and a double-blind study was indicated. Each representative of a specialty segment was engaged in a suit to support his or her own expertise. Looking on from the periphery, the psychiatrist stated that each was struggling for personal survival and vested interest. The vector forces of the various specialties were pulling away from one another.

Change is apparent in the surgical domain. There is an increasing appreciation for the capabilities and appropriateness of other therapeutic modalities. Most surgeons have expressed a preference for the use of drugs in the management of deep venous thrombosis; excision of malignancy of the breast has generally been modified so that less tissue is removed; sarcomatous limbs are now preserved with the aid of radiation and chemotherapy; and it is now almost universally appreciated that radical operations are no longer indicated for localized Hodgkin's disease. These examples should not be regarded as an expression of an attitude of conservatism versus radicalism; these terms should be deleted from the medical lexicon, since who is to say which approach is truly more conservative or more radical?

The ideal symposium and the ideal practice of medicine would have a given specialist act as devil's advocate for a therapeutic modality other than his or her own. But alas, we are all human and feel obliged to champion our own cause and the Utopia that Sir Thomas More described in 1516 will never exist.

Utopian Apparel

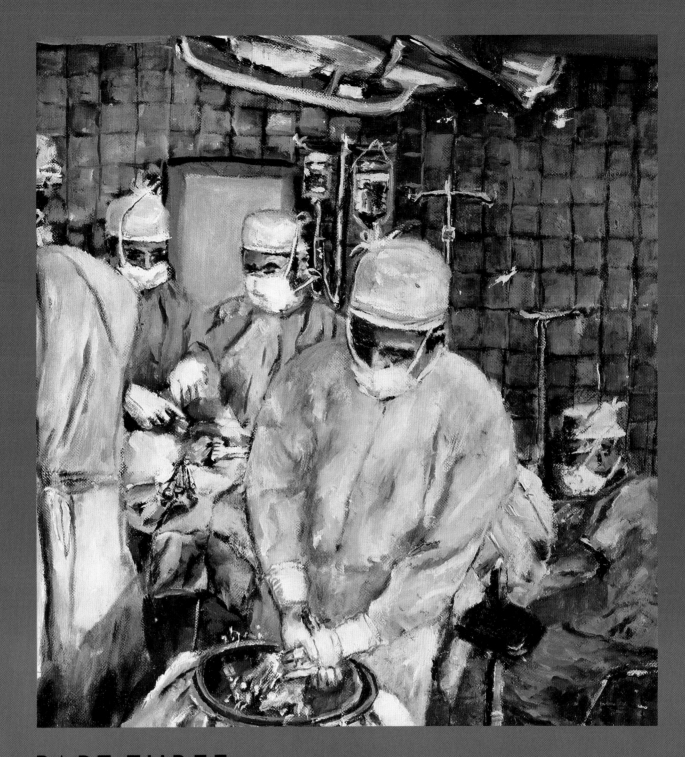

PART THREE

*The Stage
and Its Players*

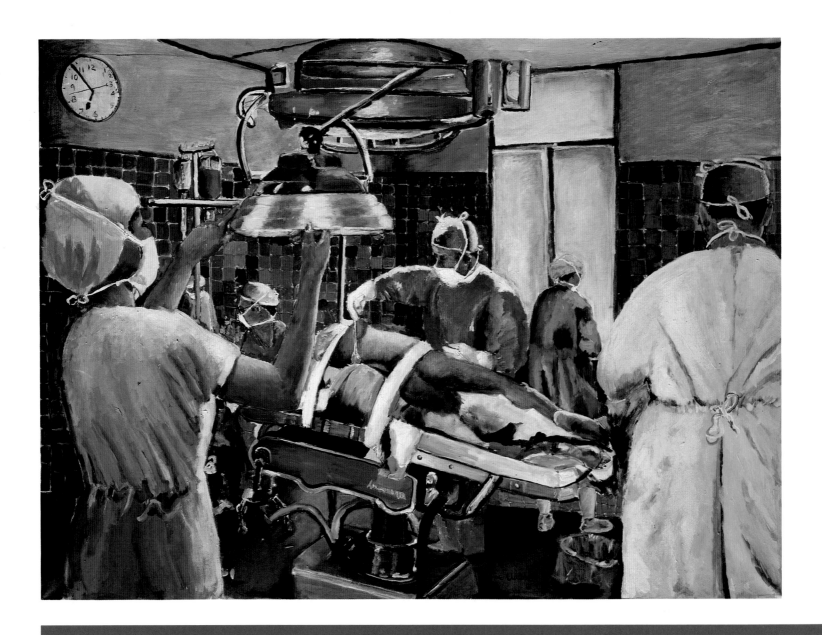

Operating Room. 1989. Oil on canvas, 60 x 66".

The modern surgical environment often expresses the ideas of mechanical, electrical, and systems analysis engineers and behavioral psychologists—occasionally producing a Tower of Babel effect. Often the specific needs of the surgeon are forgotten. Perhaps this is because the operating room has received remarkably little attention from surgeons. What follows are historical vignettes in which the operating room is dominant.

Sir Arthur Conan Doyle describes in his tale, "Round the Red Lamp," the way Lister's operating theater looked in 1872. "The operating table . . . was of unpainted deal, plain, strong, and scrupulously clean. A sheet of brown water-proofing covered half of it, and beneath stood a large tin tray full of sawdust. . . . In front of the window, there was a board . . . strewed with glittering instruments, forceps and tenacula saws, cannulas and trocars. A line of knives, with long thin, delicate blades, lay at one side."

However, J.R. Leeson, who was a house surgeon to Lister, wrote the following in *Lister As I Knew Him:* "In the centre of the worn and bloodstained room sprinkled with sawdust was the operating table, an ordinary kitchen table, devoid of any accessories. . . . The operating table looked as if it were never washed." Antedating the Listerian operating theatre are other rooms that have captured the fancy of medical historians. Sir Russell Brock chronicled the restoration of the operating theater, built in 1821, of the old St. Thomas' Hospital. When the hospital was demolished to make way for a railway, the room was reconstructed in the herb garret over the church. Forgotten in the attic, the operating room was rediscovered in 1956.

John Flint South's memorials, published in 1888, note the operating room of that day had no formal heating, plumbing, or ventilation, and pupils were packed "like herrings in a barrel, but not so quiet." In the St. Thomas operating room, anesthesia was first used in 1846. Among the many surgeons who used it was Sir Astley Cooper.

Brock contended that this was the oldest operating room extant. But Alfred R. Henderson commented on the "circular room" in the Pennsylvania Hospital, which became available both for surgery and for lectures in 1804. It adjoined America's first "recovery room." It was, in fact, the second surgical amphitheater built in America, the one in New York Hospital antedating it by 1 year. When the Pennsylvania Hospital operating room was in use, its three rows of wooden benches held about 130 students, but it was frequently overcrowded. Since 1868, it has served as a lounge for the house staff.

Appropriately, the workshop of the modern surgeon is a room, not a theater, since few observers are admitted. But the operating room is a stage for two featured players—patient and surgeon. Engineering expertise should be aimed at satisfying the needs of this pair.

The Surgical Stage

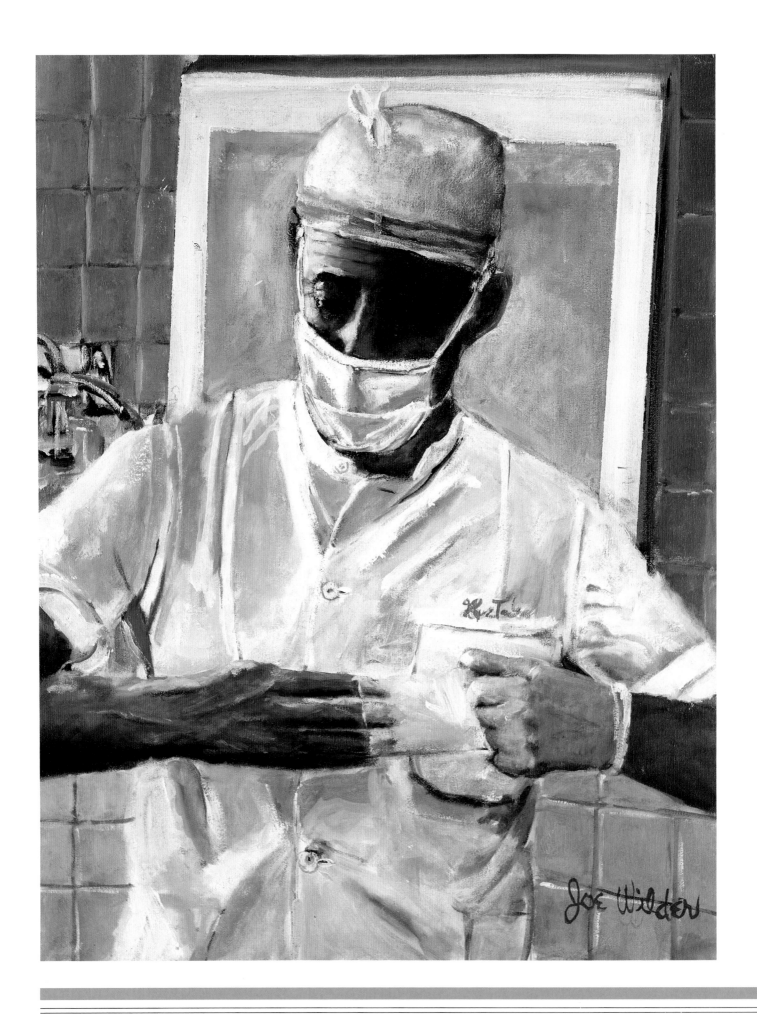

Removing Gloves. 1987. Oil on canvas, 20 x 16″.

In considering the physical characteristics of a surgeon, John Halle, in his sixteenth century translation of Lanfranc's *Chirurgia Parva*, conjured a chimeric image: "A chirurgien should have three dyvers properties in his person. That is to saie, a harte as the harte of a lyon, his eyes like the eyes of an hawke, and his handes the handes of a woman."

Sushruta, an Indian surgeon who lived sometime between the eighth and sixth centuries B.C., wrote that a physician "should be cleanly in his habits and well shaved, and should not allow his nails to grow. He should wear white garments . . . and walk about with a mild and benignant look as a friend of all created beings. . . ." A century or two later, Hippocrates indicated that "the dignity of a physician requires that he look healthy and as plump as nature intended him to be."

Oliver Wendell Holmes, in his poem entitled "Rip Van Winkle, M.D." indicated that "folks want their doctors mouldy like their cheese." A. Benson Cannon extended this thesis by stating, "It is a good thing for a physician to have prematurely gray hair and itching piles. The first makes him appear to know more than he does, and the second gives him an expression of concern which the patient interprets as being on his behalf."

There is an ancient proverb that cautioned: Beware of the young doctor and the old barber. This was paraphrased when surgery became more legitimate and on an equal footing with medicine. An Italian and French proverb insisted that a surgeon should be young and a physician old. In the first century A.D. Celsus made the same point, writing, "Now a surgeon should be youthful or at any rate nearer youth than age; with a strong and steady hand which never trembles and ready to use the left hand as well as the right. . . ." In the thirteenth century, Henri de Mondeville enunciated the physical characteristics of a good surgeon: "He should have well shaped members, especially hands with long slender fingers mobile and not tremulous." Paracelsus went so far as to specifically state that a surgeon should not have a red beard.

The truth is that images are not real; appearance is not pertinent. The true essence of the surgeon resides deep within and becomes outwardly apparent at the time of professional commitment.

Portraits of the Past

49

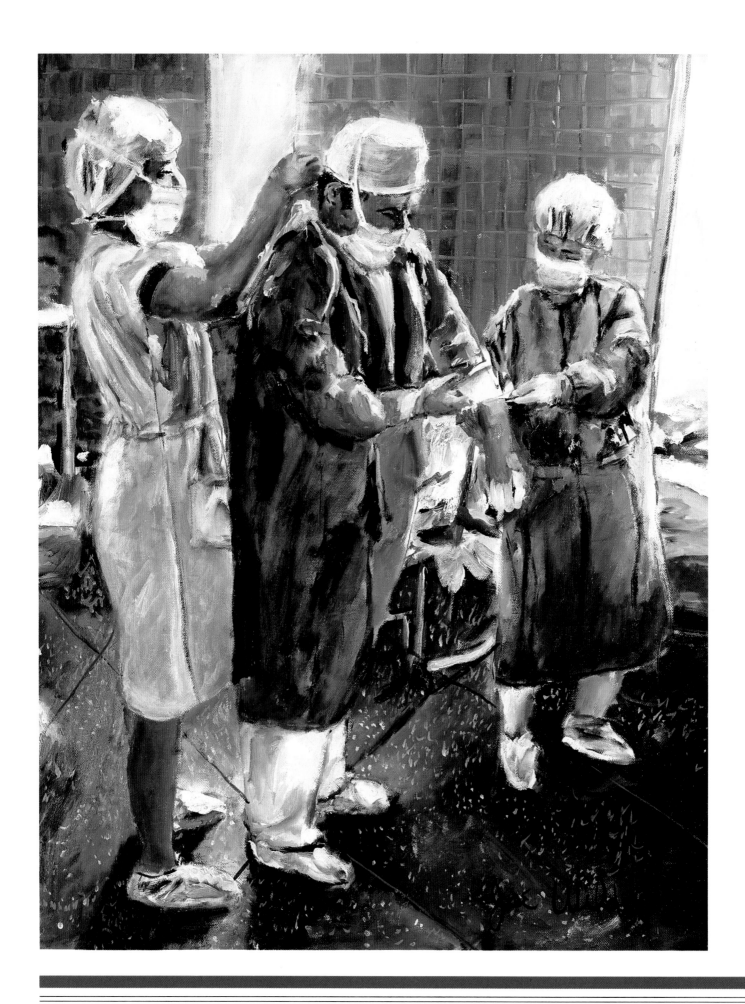

Gowned and Gloved. 1987. Oil on canvas, 18 x 14″.

Is the *ken* mightier than the sword? When today's practicing surgeons and their surgical progenitors are compared, an evolutionary process is apparent. The first phase of this process emphasized the technical and mechanical expansion of the art—the establishment of a competent, dextrous "surgical *Homo manualis.*" After more structures and organs could be removed and repaired with increased safety related to growing technical proficiency, the second evolutionary phase occurred: the development of a "surgical *Homo sapiens,*" intellectually interested in improving the patients' lot. This is a more recent and continuing event.

Today's surgeon freely converses with his nonsurgical confreres with a sense of scientific maturity and parity. It is accepted that surgeons have made many significant contributions in microbiology, physiology, immunology, and other sciences. The modern surgeon will never revert to the technical brute who was regarded as the mechanical arm of the medical profession.

The "technical brute," however, must persist if the surgeon is to maintain an appropriate role. The modern surgeon should not be apologetic for the manual aspect of his or her composite personality. In fact, it is the surgeon's *raison d'etre* in the scheme of health care delivery. The surgeon's technical capabilities constitute his or her unique contribution to therapeutics. A surgical procedure may be considered a medication, with indications, contraindications, dosage, and adverse reactions. The physician prescribes a drug, which generally a pharmacologist discovered, a pharmaceutical house modified, and a pharmacist dispenses. In an analogy, the surgeon's contributions are all inclusive. He or she advises an operation that is based on a scientific principle generally developed by a surgeon, that uses a technique devised and modified by surgeons, and that is dispensed only by surgeons. Thus, if performance is considered in an anatomic context, the surgeon is, in fact, the true therapeutic internist. To keep in tune with the times, the surgeon requires continued exposure to a harmonious atmosphere in which the opus has three themes—a scientific base, solid technique, and continued analysis.

Muscle and Mind

51

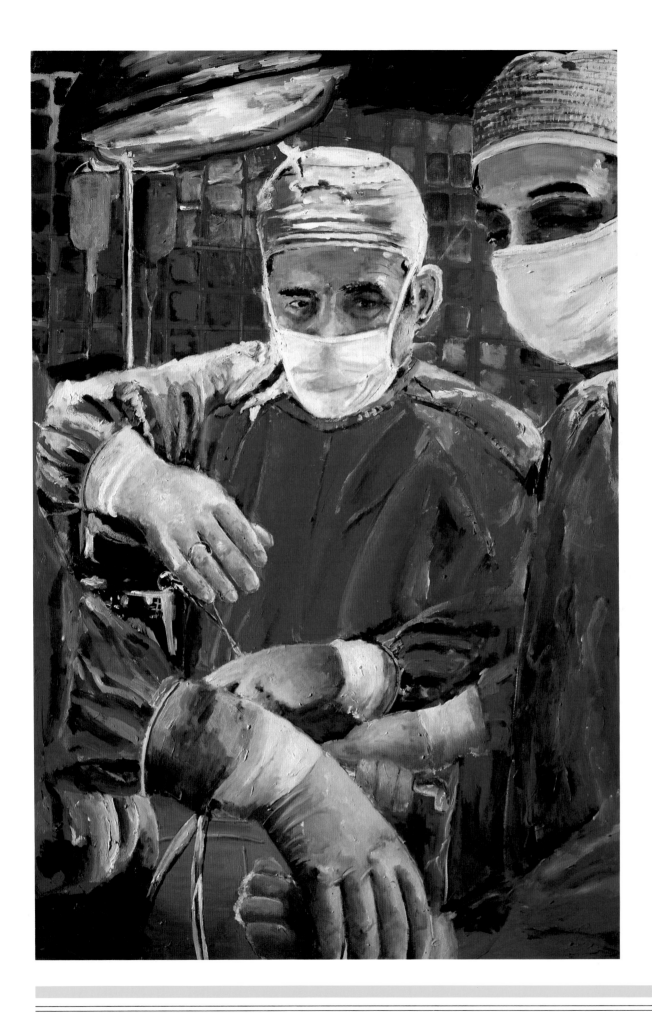

Magic Hands. 1990. Acrylic on canvas, 72 x 48″.

Mastery of surgery mandates technical skill. Lord Joseph Lister stated, "To intrude an unskilled hand into such a piece of divine mechanism as the human body is indeed a fearful responsibility." Stressing surgical technique should strike a chord for most readers, because academicians, attending physicians in community hospitals, and senior residents all are responsible in one way or another for teaching younger surgeons. This provides an opportunity for me to joust with two of my own surgical heroes with whom I disagree along these very lines. Harvey Cushing, a superb technical surgeon, wrote in 1911, "I would like to see the day when somebody would be appointed surgeon somewhere who had no hands, for the operative part is the least part of the work." And in 1978 Owen H. Wangensteen wrote that the question, "But can he operate?" should cease to be the predominant consideration of medical schools and their search committees seeking a promising future surgical leader.

I would agree that a teacher need not be the most facile surgeon, but he must be able to operate well, and he must remain an active clinician to command the respect of those whose education he shepherds. A surgical procedure, the therapeutic modality for which the surgeon is uniquely qualified, requires emphasis, appreciation, and constant nurturing. By the very nature of the field, the teaching of surgery is basically preceptorial, and the dialogue between teacher and learner should concentrate on what is not expressed as printed words in books but rather on the result of experience. As good judgment is most frequently based on vivid experiences with bad judgment, the textbook and didactic discourse cannot substitute for this experience.

The surgeon must be a virtuoso if one regards the *Oxford English Dictionary* definition of the term, "learned and skillful." The word "surgeon" literally means one who works with the hands. A surgeon must have hands that respond to the head and must be able to operate well. William D. Haggard, a professor of surgery at Vanderbilt, wrote in his book, *Surgery, Queen of the Arts*, "In the other fine arts, art is justified for the sake of art. In surgery it is a real need because upon the finesse and perfection of its artistry, the success of the surgical procedure largely and sometimes entirely depends. It is the art of the sculptor rendered with the heroism and skill of a lifesaver."

The Skill of a Lifesaver

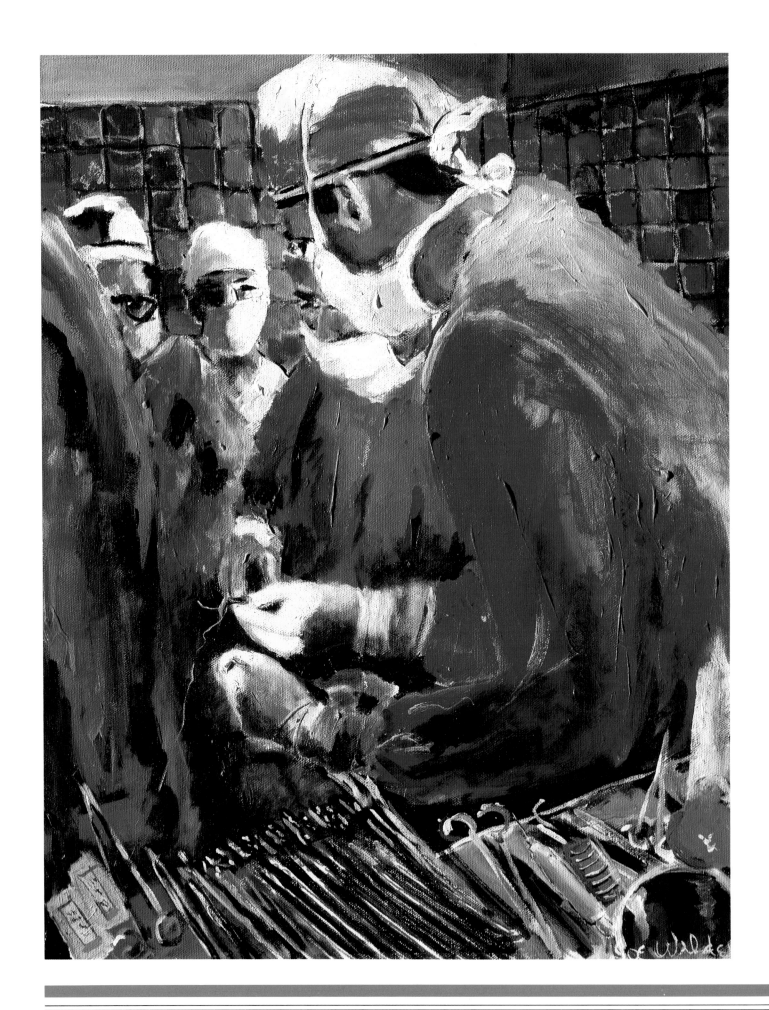

Adjusting Needle Holder. 1987. Oil on canvas, 20 x 16″.

A line from Shakespeare's *Love's Labours Lost* is, "He draweth out the thread of his verbosity finer than the staple of his argument," thus drawing a comparison between thread and staple. These two items, one old and one new, perform the same function: approximation of tissue.

The currently used stapling devices are actually elegantly engineered analogues of ancient ants. As Guido Majno points out in *The Healing Hand,* Sushruta mentions the use of the clasping jaws of ants for closing intestinal wounds. Majno also tells of a species of ants that builds its nests by temporarily stapling leaves together with their jaws and then permanently joining them by sewing using larvae with specially developed silk glands. This suggests that even ants may find it appropriate to avoid a unilateral approach to a given problem.

About 4000 years ago, the first use of skin-closure strips was documented in the Edwin Smith Papyrus. In 30 A.D., Celsus described small metal clips, similar to the modern Michel clip. About 120 years later, Galen wrote that sutures should be made of materials that do not rot easily; he suggested silk, when obtainable. Catgut, he indicated, would also be appropriate because of its strength and availability from musicians (the name derives from *kitgut,* the "kit" being an early form of strung musical instrument); he did not appreciate catgut's absorbability. Rhazes in 900 A.D. and Albucassis during the following century advocated using sutures made from sheep intestines. About the same time, Avicenna preached that in the presence of infection, linen thread should not be used, since it tends to break down, and advised that pig bristle be used in such circumstances, thus providing a mention of the first monofilament suture. Philip Syng Physick conducted the first experiments with absorbable sutures, successfully employing buckskin and kidskin, and noted little success with catgut, which he felt did not dissolve sufficiently. In 1858, Sims, with some bravado, suggested that the silver ligature was "the major surgical achievement of the nineteenth century." Lister, an early disciple of Sims, went on to develop antiseptic catgut and later tanned it with chromic acid to delay absorption. In the 1880s, Kocher strongly advocated silk, which had as its major champion Halsted, whose classic paper on this appeared in 1913. Advances in technology are responsible for more recent changes. In Britain and the United States they have led to the development of a variety of synthetic monofilament sutures. And Russian technology has brought us the staple.

A lesson learned from the ants is that more than one approach may be used solely or adjunctively. For those who prefer to adhere solely to the time-honored techniques, Augustin Belloste's line, published in *Suite du Chirurgiens d'hôpital* in 1733, should be considered: "That which is New at this time will one day be Ancient; as what is Ancient was once New. It is not the length of time which can give Value to Things, it is their own Excellency."

Twixt Thread and Staple

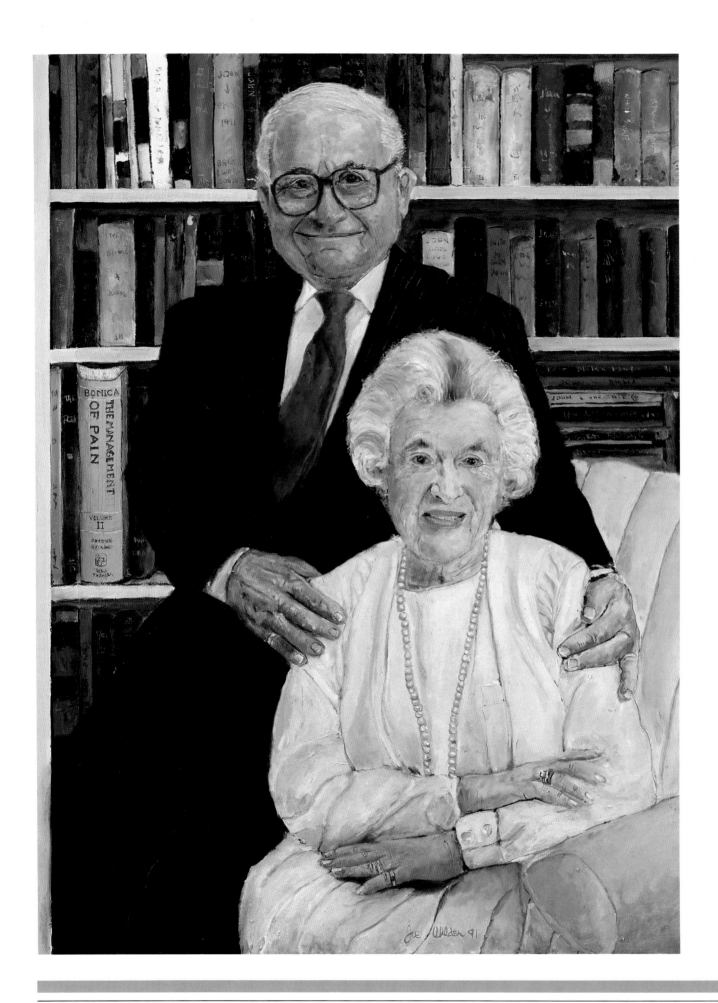

Dr. and Mrs. John Bonica. 1991. Oil on canvas, 48 x 36″. Collection Dr. and Mrs. John Bonica.

Be not overcome of evil, but overcome evil with good—*Romans XII, 21.* St. Augustine stated, "The greatest evil is physical pain." Because surgeons by their craft inevitably and unavoidably inflict pain on their patients, amelioration and control of pain are integral to the management of these patients.

Effective drugs for the control of pain have been available for many years, but during those years surgery patients have continued to suffer needlessly as a consequence of inadequate medications. Nursing care does not focus on the control of pain; all too often, ordered drugs are not administered in a timely fashion. Surgeons, and particularly younger surgery residents, are frequently negligent in anticipating and appreciating postoperative pain. Samuel Johnson said, "Those who do not feel pain seldom think that it is felt."

Pain is a constant sequitur of a surgical procedure, but it can be blunted, or, preferably, erased. Sir Charles Illingworth, the great Scottish professor of surgery who trained many of the modern surgical leaders in the United Kingdom, waxed eloquent in his consideration of pain: "Every sentient being knows what is meant by pain but the true significance of pain eludes the most sapient. For philosophers, pain is a problem of metaphysics, and an exercise for stoics; for mystics it is an ecstacy, for the religious, a travail meekly to be borne, for clinicians a symptom to be understood and an ill to be relieved."

"Pain" derives from the Latin word *poena,* meaning punishment. The endurance of postoperative pain by patients is truly an uncalled for punishment, particularly in a time when patient-controlled analgesia and continuous epidural analgesia are available. There should be no contest to determine how *little* medication is needed, and rarely is there a concern that addiction will result. The potential for pain must be anticipated and addressed prospectively. The patient's assessment of experienced pain should be accepted and responded to immediately. Peter Mere Latham, physician and teacher of medicine in early nineteenth century England, wrote, "Not only degrees of pain, but its existence, in any degree, must be taken upon testimony of the patient."

Simply stated, the endurance of pain should not be regarded as an obligatory component of recovery from an operation. Part of the ethical conduct of a physician must be directed toward the effective control of patient pain. As John Milton stated in *Paradise Lost:*

But Pain Is Perfect Miserie,
The Worst of Evils,
And Excessive, Overturnes
All Patience.

Punishment Is Crime

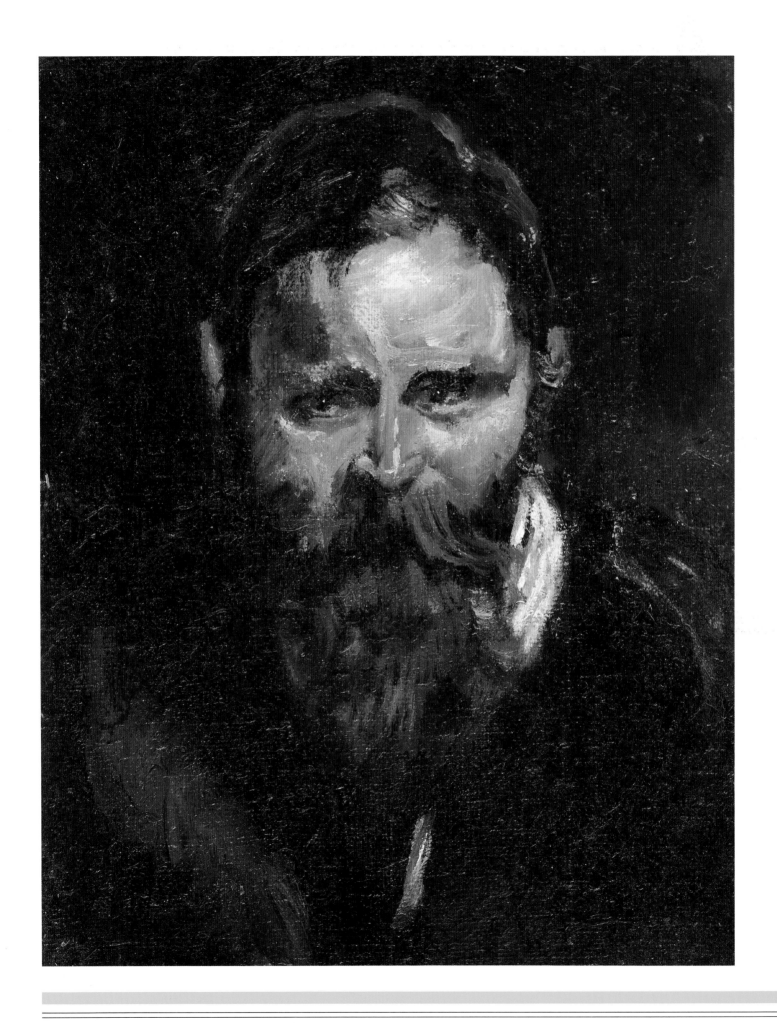

Philosopher, after Rubens. 1988. Oil on panel, 7½ x 6″.

As chief resident in surgery, I had the opportunity to select the annual visiting professor for our institution. My choice of Dr. Dragstedt was based on many factors. He was highly regarded as an outstanding researcher whose contributions had far-reaching clinical application, as a surgeon, as a revered teacher, and as an administrator of an esteemed department of surgery—a Renaissance man thriving in an age of specialization.

Today an atmosphere antithetical to Renaissance ideals pervades, and these questions arise: "What compromises must our surgical leaders make?" and "What priorities must persist?"

The major encroachment on the Renaissance concept has been the exponential growth and complexity of administrative demands, locally and nationally. Administration is essentially incompatible with academia. As Paul Goodman wrote in his *Community of Scholars:* "It is the genius of administrators to enforce a false harmony in a situation that should be rife with conflict."

In many regards, the Renaissance personality continues to characterize surgical leaders. These individuals, more than other members of the higher echelon of the academic community, have resisted transformation by administrative requirements. Teaching is considered the major function. Research can be done in research institutes; clinical surgery is performed with equivalent excellence in many hospitals outside the academic sphere. The academic surgeon's prime responsibility is the education of medical students and residents.

It is fortunate for our future that good people must teach. The teaching process is an indispensable creative stimulus for scholar and scientist. Nothing is more erroneous than the cliché: "Those who can, do; those who can't, teach." As John Rice stated, "Teaching is a secondary art. A man is a good teacher if he is a better something else; for teaching is communication and has a better something else as the storehouse of things to be communicated." It is therefore essential that the academic surgeon maintain the posture of a clinical surgeon and at least the attitude of a researcher, if not a continued interest in investigation.

Some change is inevitable. Just as the Renaissance period in art gave way to the school of Mannerism, with artists adopting some methods of their predecessors but producing a unique effect, surgical leadership will undergo stylistic alterations. A direct approach and independent action, however, will continue to set surgical leaders apart as much-needed mavericks in the academic community. Departments of surgery will be administered and national commitments met in an appropriate manner, similar to that which surgeons use in ministering to sick patients. Thus, the priorities that will persist are patient care, scientific inquiry, and dissemination of information.

Revival of the Renaissance

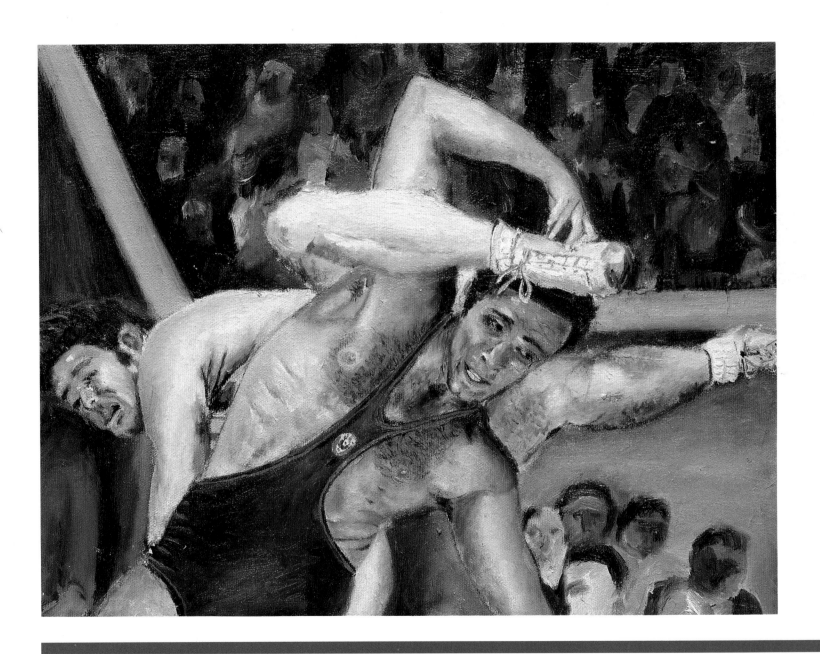

Scissors-Hold. 1984. Oil on canvas, 12 x 16″.

Physicians and surgeons have an appreciation of a common goal that found expression as far back as the Hippocratic era in this aphorism: "In practice as in honor, medicine and surgery are one." Plutarch wrote, "Internists are seldom jealous of surgeons; nay, they back up and recommend one another." Up to the time of Avicenna, surgery was seen as an alternative way to treat disease the physician could reach with his hand.

The split between medicine and surgery had its roots in clerical, feudal, and humanistic conceits. The Rheims (1125) and Lateran (1139) councils restricted surgery by clerics. At Tours, surgery's academic death knell, "Ecclesia abbhoret a sanguine," was first heard. In the twelfth century the University of Paris excluded all who worked with their hands, expelling surgery from the liberal arts.

Reparation of this schism was analogous to neuronal repair: It began centrally and progressed slowly. One of the most quoted comments of the time was Lanfranc's in *Chirurgia Magna* in 1296: "Oh Lord, why is there such great difference between surgeons and physicians? . . . No man can be a good physician who knows no surgery; and conversely, no one can be a good surgeon without knowledge of medicine." Guy de Chauliac, regarded as the founder of modern surgical doctrine in Western Europe, claimed surgery was medicine's co-equal; Henri de Mondeville more appropriately stated, "Surgery is but a method of treatment. It belongs to all of medicine."

In 1904, Sir T. Clifford Allbutt, Regius Professor of Physic at Oxford, promoted the idea that medicine had benefited significantly from its connection with surgery. Certainly, all physicians appreciated the contributions of surgical studies of the anatomy. The French, extending the political precept of "égalité" to medicine, abolished separate schools for doctors and surgeons and the external distinctions between the disciplines. Other countries followed suit.

The end of polarity resulted primarily from changes in surgeons' attitudes, reflected in the great John Hunter's statement: "This last part of surgery, namely operations, is a reflection of the healing art; it is a test of acknowledgement of the insufficiency of surgery. It is like an armed savage who attempts to get by force what civilized man would get by stratagem." The great physician René Laënnec praised surgical contributions: "In one word, I have tried, with regard to diagnosis, to put internal organic lesions on the same level as surgical diseases."

The successful symbiotic existence of surgeon and physician has led to experiments in interdisciplinary teaching and the founding of associations where the two groups can meet. The establishment of such disciplines as dermatology and gynecology, in which the physician governs pharmacologic and surgical management, may presage the future management of other organ systems.

Symbiosis

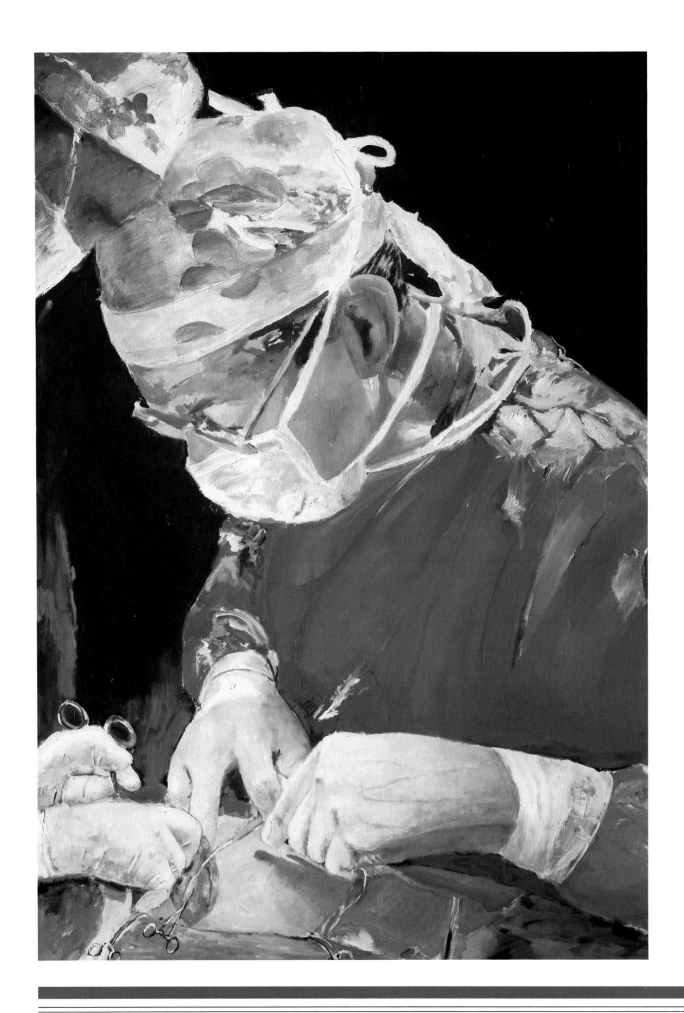

Chief of Surgery. 1990. Acrylic on canvas, 61 x 42″. Collection Cathy Karlin.

In 1925 Evarts Graham wrote that in addition to its great artists, "at the present time . . . surgery needs more men of the composer type." Over the ensuing years, surgical science and genius have been responsible for new therapeutic scores and themes. The requisite artistry and inventiveness of surgeons must now be joined metaphorically by orchestration and conduction as we consider the new role that the modern surgeon must assume.

Angiographic control of bleeding is but one sign of the time—a time characterized by an ever-increasing number of nonsurgical procedures that may effectively manage disorders previously restricted therapeutically to the surgical domain. To this specific example could be added dilation of stenosed arteries; dilation, drainage, and stenting of the biliary tract; ultrasonographically or computer tomographically directed drainage of intraperitoneal abscesses and cysts; biopsy of hepatic, pancreatic, and retroperitoneal tumors; and percutaneous fragmentation of renal stones. Invoking another set of nonsurgical players, we could include endoscopic treatment of mucosal or variceal bleeding, sphincterotomy, and endoscopic removal of polyps.

Acting as a conductor who must draw the best from various artists and meld them to produce optimal therapy, the surgeon must appreciate the relative applicability of a variety of therapeutic interventions, including the operation itself, and select without vested interest what is preferable for a given patient.

Certain aphorisms pertain to the surgeon's decision-making role and the selection of the most appropriate modality. Before becoming overly enthusiastic about a new therapeutic approach, Alfred Blalock wrote, "It usually requires a considerable time to determine with certainty the virtues of a new method of treatment and usually still longer to ascertain the harmful effects." The virtuoso surgeon playing the role of conductor must be introspective and counter personal vested interests. Von Langenbeck wrote, "It is less important to invent new operations and new techniques of operating than to find ways and means to avoid surgery." And Robert Tuttle Morris emphasized that "the greatest triumph of surgery today . . . lies in finding ways of avoiding surgery."

The surgeon is well prepared to orchestrate and to conduct virtuosos from various disciplines in the therapeutic ensemble. The surgeon is the one player who is totally familiar with and therefore appreciates the ultimate therapy of an operative procedure. The surgeon is the one therapeutic performer who has a continuous, extensive dialogue with the patient and is held in unique esteem by the patient. By virtue of these postures, the modern surgeon is eminently qualified to direct the regimen and must therefore wield not only the scalpel but also the baton.

Scalpel and Baton

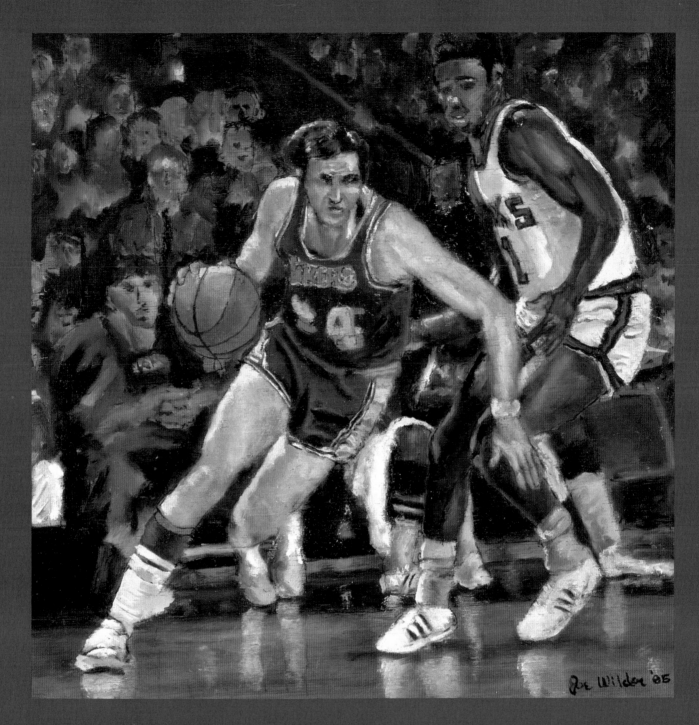

PART FOUR

Heroes

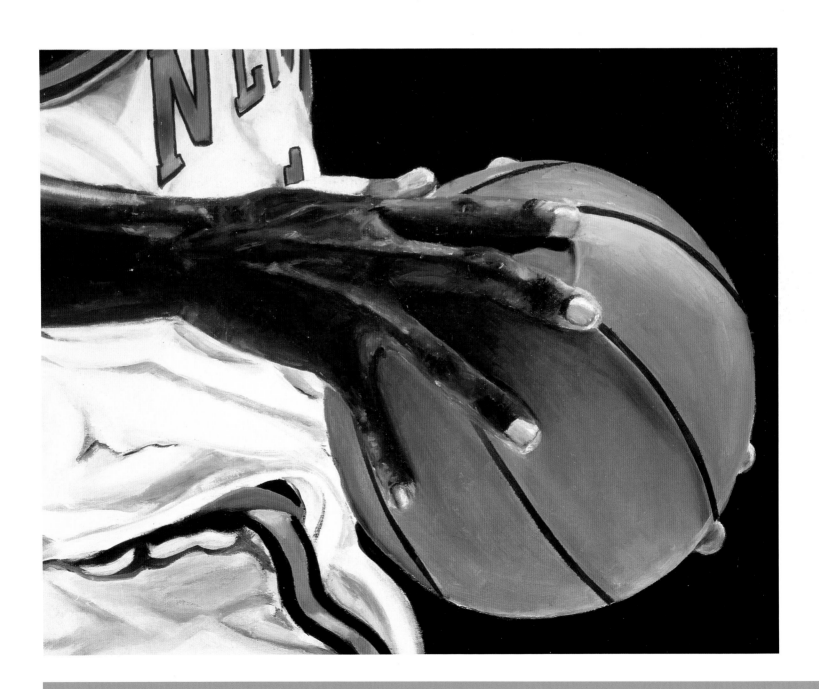

Detail of Willis Reed. 1975.

Recently, driving on the Autostrada to Florence from the west, I passed a sign for the city of Lucca, the name associated with Ugo (Hugo), the first surgeon to challenge the Galenic doctrine that pus is an essential prelude to wound healing, and therefore "laudable." Ugo de Burgogna, a great teacher, never published, but is immortalized in the writings of his disciple—who may well have been his son—Theodoric, Bishop of Cervia.

In Theodoric's *Chirurgia*, written in 1267, and published in 1498, he stressed at the onset that the word "surgery" derives from *cheiros,* meaning hand, and *ourgia,* action. In the introduction to the book, the essence of surgical education is spelled out: "It behooves practitioners of surgery to frequent the places where skilled surgeons operate, and to attend these operations diligently and commit them to memory." This is followed by an enunciation of what we modern surgeons have referred to as Halstedian principles: "There is no need . . . to be rash or daring, but let them be foresighted, gentle and circumspect, in order that with the greatest deliberateness and gentleness they may operate under all circumstances with what gentleness they can, especially around cerebral membranes, sensitive parts and other ticklish places."

The text chronicles one of Hugo's great contributions—the demonstration that healing per primam was desirable and attainable. Theodoric's writings also parallel the Edwin Smith Papyrus in declaring that some patients cannot be treated. "Therefore before you proceed to the treatment of the patient, consider his symptoms, and if what you see is obviously bad and likely to worsen, leave him alone." But the greatest contribution of the text that led the English physician, Sir Clifford Albutt, to regard Theodoric as the most original surgeon of his time, was Theodoric's role as a pioneer in the field of dry aseptic surgery. In *Chirurgia* it is written:

> For it is not necessary, as Roger and Roland have written, as many of their disciples teach, and as all modern surgeons profess, that pus should be generated in wounds. No error can be greater than this. Such a practice is indeed to hinder Nature, to prolong the disease and to prevent the conglutination and consolidation of the wound.

In the Dark Ages two beacons—Hugo and Theodoric—shined, but their light was snuffed out for 6 centuries until Listerian luminescence had its effect.

Two Beacons in the Dark

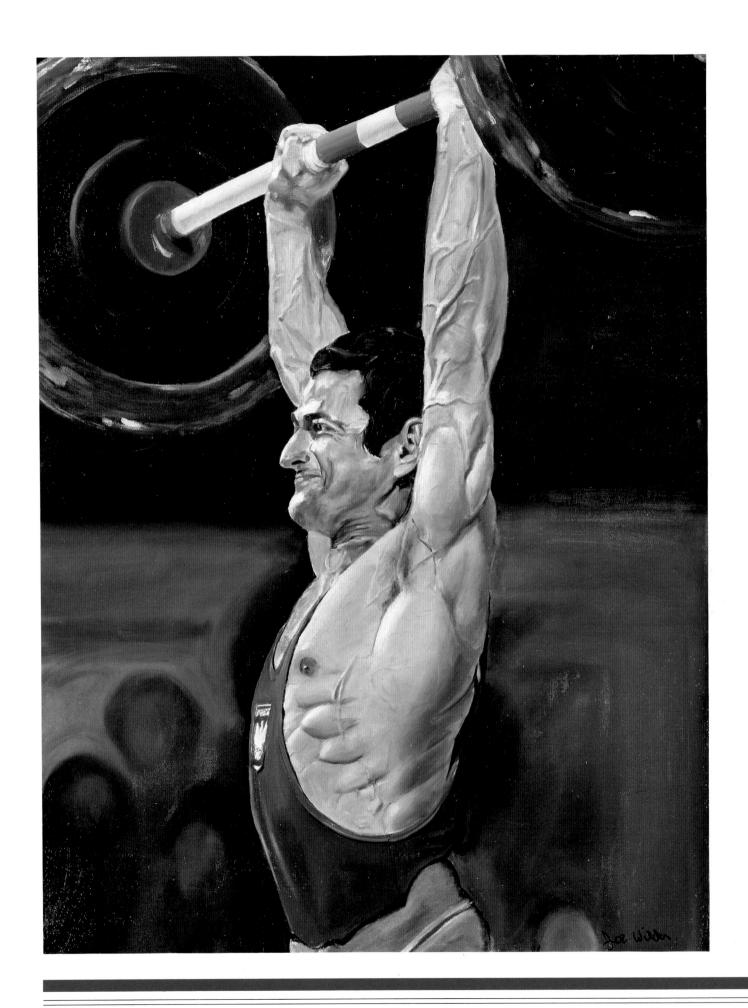

Smalcerz: Fly-Weight Lifting Champion. 1976. Oil on canvas, 30 x 28″. Collection Morris W. Offit.

*H*ow would a membership committee of an elite organization or a peer review panel react today to Leonardo da Vinci, a man who was illegitimate, did not publish his scientific work, and divided his interest among at least six fields including anatomy, architecture, engineering, music, sculpture, and painting? What would be the critical assessment of a painter who produced fewer than ten major pieces and who erred in selecting the material to be used for his grand fresco, dooming "The Last Supper" to self-destruction?

What would be the response to an inventor whose inventions would have to await a later age to reach fruition? Would the contemporary critics admit that the anatomic drawings of our subject, including those derivative of medieval predecessors, those resulting from observation and dissection of more than 30 bodies, and those applying physical laws to the human body, were the ultimate synthesis of art and science?

Would the members of the establishment envy a man whose intellect was matched by his physical attributes? Would the authorities be swayed or have their personal pride tweaked by our subject's diatribes, as exemplified by the following:

Many will think that they can with reason blame me, alleging that my proofs are contrary to the authority of certain men held in great reverence by their unexperienced judgments, not considering that my works are the issue of simple and plain experience which is the true mistress.

Should not the established authorities of all ages accept the fact that many truths will be proved false, and aphorisms are better set in sand than in stone, and that the maverick of the present will contribute to the development of a new mean and a new credo for the future?

Consider the Maverick

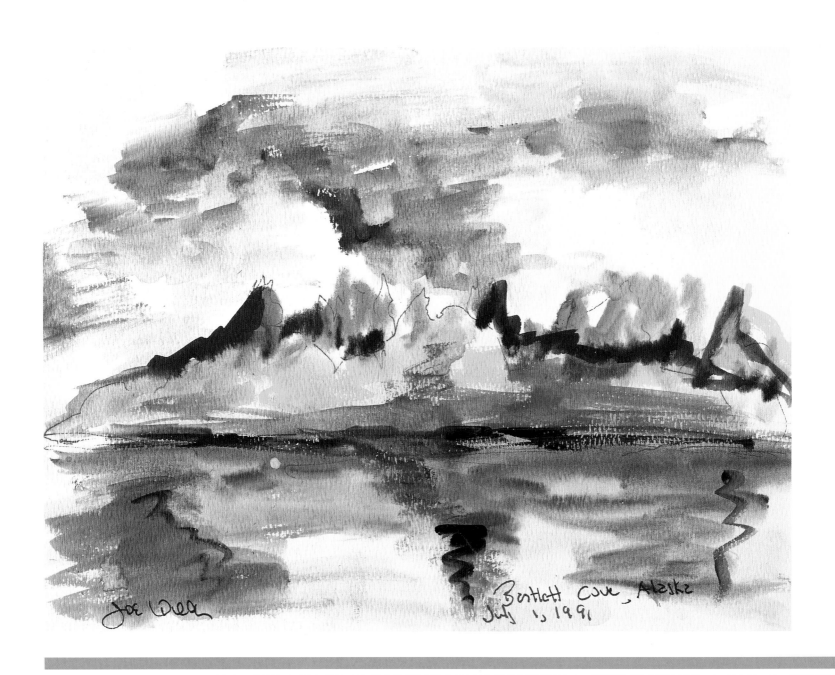

Bartlett Cove, Alaska. 1991. Watercolor, 9 x 12″.

The Treaty of Paris defined the boundaries of the United States. The map used by the commissioners who negotiated the treaty was made by a member of the medical profession who merits our recognition. John Mitchell was born on April 13, 1771, in Lancaster County, Virginia, educated in Edinburgh as a student of Alexander Munro Primus, and returned to practice medicine in Urbana, Virginia.

As Theodore Hornberger, the author of *The Scientific Ideas of John Mitchell,* wrote, "Few men rival Mitchell as a key to the problems of the intellectual life of the colonies. He has a place in the early history of American botany, zoology, physiology, medicine, cartography, climatology, and agriculture, to say nothing of politics. He was for a time perhaps the ablest scientific investigator in North America, and is credited both with the authorship of the earliest work on the principles of taxonomy to be written in what is now the United States, and with making of what has been called the most important map in American history."

John Mitchell was an avid botanist who contributed to Linnaeus' *Species Plantarum;* in this work, the partridgeberry honored the Virginia physician with the name *Mitchella repens*. This Virginia physician was also the first to dissect the opossum, and reported his findings in 1745 in what some regard as the first entry into zoologic literature from North America. Mitchell's first publication, which previously had appeared in the *Philosophical Transactions of the Royal Society,* considered the causes of different pigmentations of "Negroes." The author concluded that both the white and black man descended from the same parents and that color did not represent a "black humor or fluid parts in the skin." As a physician, he was regarded as an early authority on what was thought to be yellow fever. As an intellectual, he was sufficiently regarded to become a member of the American Philosophical Society.

In 1745, Mitchell left for England because of ill health and did not continue his practice of medicine. In 1750, he apparently had drawn a map to delineate British and French claims in North America. This document has never been uncovered. In 1755, using fresh sources of information that were sent to him directly from the governor's surveyors in the colonies, Mitchell drew his famous map. Fifteen years after his death, Mitchell's map was used as the prime document to establish boundaries at the end of the American Revolution. Its value as an authoritative document continued well into the twentieth century, when it was used as evidence in boundary disputes between Canada and Newfoundland, Wisconsin and Michigan, and New Jersey and Delaware.

Except for this single document, John Mitchell made no great scientific contribution, yet few have been as versatile as this native American, who was regarded by the famous American botanist, John Bartram, as "an ingenious man."

Defining Boundaries

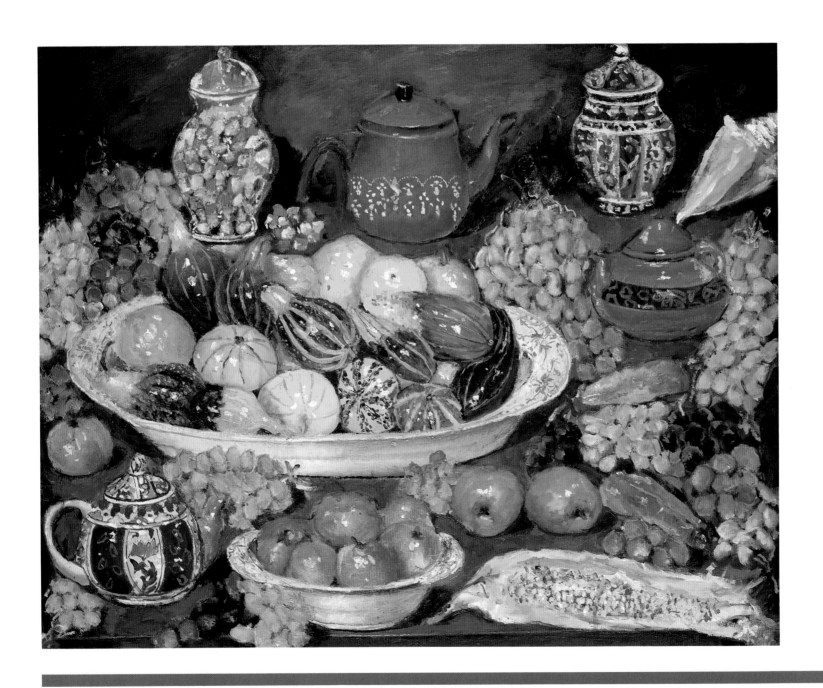

Thanksgiving. 1992. Oil on canvas, 24 x 30″.

*T*hanksgiving is a holiday that is unique to the United States. Even the date on which we commemorate the Pilgrims' expression of thanks for survival is a governmental fiat. It is reasonable, at a time of national holiday, to pay tribute to a great American surgeon who was associated with many firsts in the history of our country.

Born in Long Island in 1729, a student of William Hunter and the recipient of the degree of Doctor of Medicine from the University of Rheims in 1751, John Jones came to be regarded as the most skillful surgeon in New York; his reputation was enhanced when he performed the first successful lithotomy in this country. He was a major force behind the establishment of the first medical school in the colonies and became the first Professor of Surgery when Kings College (later Columbia University College of Physicians and Surgeons) was granted its charter in 1767. Four years later he actively contributed to the founding of the New York Hospital, the first hospital in that city and second only to the Pennsylvania Hospital in the colonies.

Dr. Jones's words were as important as his deeds, and his 1755 book, *Plain Concise Practical Remarks on the Treatment of Wounds and Fractures,* was the first medical book published in the colonies. Modern deans could pay heed to his writings regarding the importance of surgery in a general medical education:

> This ancient branch of medicine call'd Surgery, according to the strict grammatical meaning of the word, signified manual operation, but the science & art of surgery, tho' more clear & certain in its objects, than that of Physic, is equally various, extensive & difficult of attainment. And I have ever been of opinion that young Physicians might lay the foundation for medical knowledge, by an attentive observation of those disorders, which surgery presented to their view . . .

In his introductory lecture to his course in surgery Dr. Jones offered sage advice about the preparation of a surgeon when he stated:

> The mind . . . must be prepar'd before its entrance into the study of surgery by a previous acquisition of those branches of knowledge, which form the rules by which we ought to conduct ourselves in the cure of diseases. 'Tis to such cultivated geniuses, that surgery owes its greatest progress—such were a Serverinus, a Fallopius, a Hildanus, a Vesalius, a Scultetus, a Le Dran, a Wiseman, a Cheselden, a Monro, a Sharp. These illustrious surgeons, whose minds were prepar'd by the study of the learn'd languages, cultivated by the belles lettres, and enrich'd with the knowledge of Philosophy, have hung up the best lights to conduct us through the dark and intricate windings of our art.

John Jones deserves a position of primacy on the chronologic list of American surgical heroes, and surgical personalities justly should be considered heroes as stated by Ralph Waldo Emerson, "In the hands of the discoverer medicine becomes a heroic art. . . . Where life is dear he is a demigod."

Keeping Up With a Jones

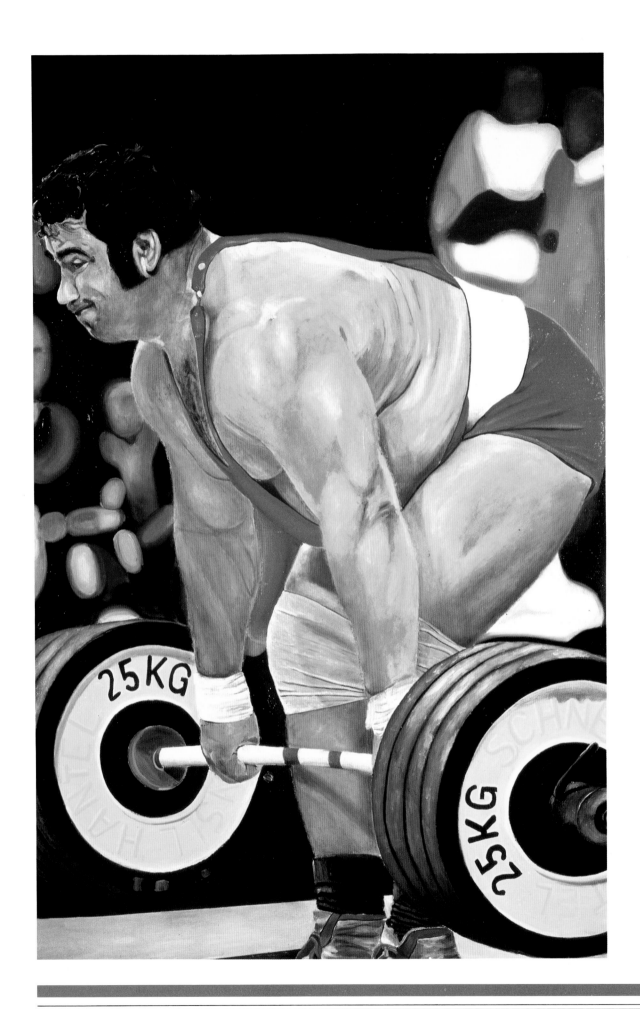

Alexeev, World's Strongest Man. 1975. Oil on canvas, 64 x 42″. Collection Mr. and Mrs. Wallace Friedman.

On July 14, 1789, with the storming of the Bastille, the curtain was raised on the drama of the French Revolution. The leader of the 1500 students at the forefront of the storming crowd was a 23-year-old, born July 8, 1766, who was to become the greatest military surgeon of the time.

Dominique Jean Larrey was the first military surgeon to be formally acknowledged by his government and was referred to as one "whose indefatigable care of the wounded eased the suffering of mankind, on such a day, served the cause of humanity itself, and contributed to saving the gallant defenders of our country." This accolade was bestowed in the pre-Napoleonic period when Larrey tended the Army of the Rhine that was fighting the King of Prussia and the Emperor of Austria as they attempted to rescue their royal brother. At a time in 1791 when the famous battle hymn that began "Allons enfants de la patrie, Le jour de gloire est arrivé" was penned, Larrey introduced the "flying ambulance" drawn by two or four horses to carry the injured to safety, and he advocated early amputation to reduce the incidence of infection and gangrene.

It was the same Larrey of aggressive amputation fame, using three circular cuts at sequentially higher levels during a 2-minute period to provide a good stump, who dedicated himself to preserving limbs whenever possible. His humanism and ethics are manifest in his dictum, "We will always start with the most dangerously injured without regard to rank and distinction."

It was Larrey, surgeon to Napoleon's Imperial Guard, who in 1803 took the first recertification examination when the First Consul restored medical facilities. It was Larrey who personally performed 200 amputations in a 24-hour period during the Battle of Bordino (Moskova) on the Russian front. During the same battle he was able to preserve many limbs, including the arm of General Pajol, who sustained a comminuted fracture of the forearm.

Napoleon singled out Larrey with the summary statement, "the most virtuous man I have known." The name Larrey, whom Dupuytren regarded as "a connecting link between surgery of the last age and that of present day," is inscribed on the Arc de Triomphe in Paris and in the annals of surgery.

A Strong Link

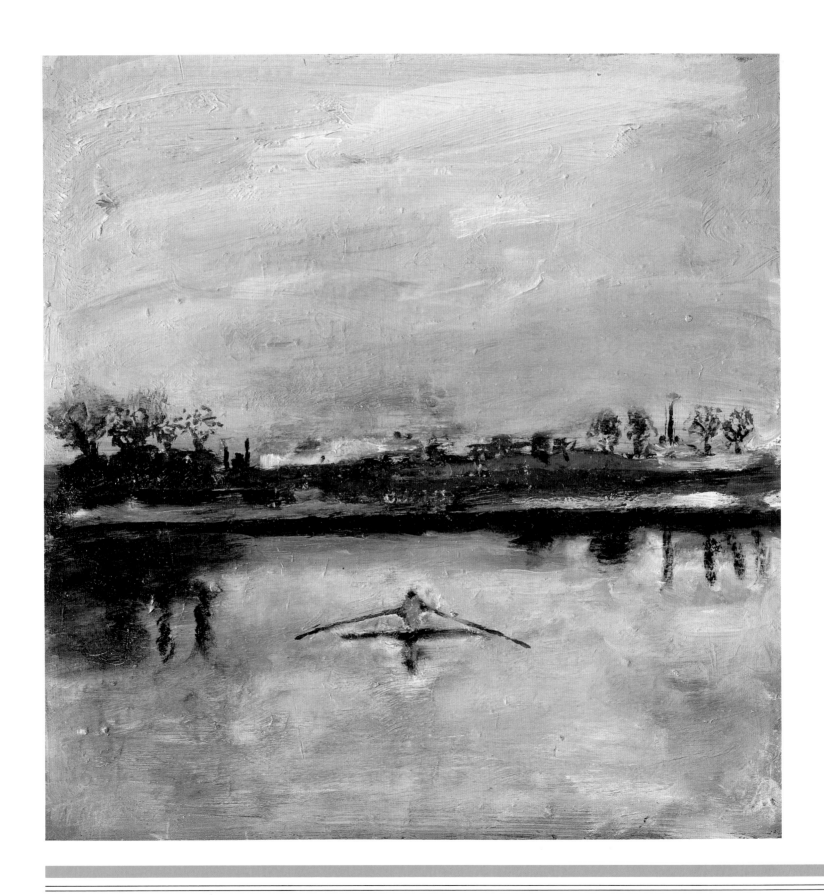

Lonely Sculler, based on Ken Robbins' photograph. 1991. Oil on panel, 8 x 8″.

An extraordinary surgeon's eclectic interests and innovative incursions earned him the title of Father of Arterial Surgery. Sir Astley Paston Cooper, Baronet (1768-1841), was a pupil of John Hunter who became Demonstrator of Anatomy of St. Thomas's Hospital at the age of 21. It is said that he did dissections almost every day of his medical life, even paying large fees to body snatchers.

The scope and depth of his contributions were truly extraordinary. In 1802 he received the Copley medal for his work on perforating the tympanic membrane for deafness resulting from obstruction of the eustachian tube. From 1804 to 1807 he wrote extensively on hernia, in 1822 on fractures and injuries of joints, in 1830 on diseases of the testes, in 1832 on the anatomy of the thymus gland, and in 1840 on the breast. The eponyms of Cooper's ligament in the inguinal region, Cooper's suspensory ligament of the breast, and Cooper's (retroperitoneal) hernia still exist.

His deserved claim to Father of Arterial Surgery has both experimental and clinical bases. Experimentally in the dog he showed that both carotid arteries could be ligated with impunity and that ligation of the abdominal aorta of the dog was associated with survival but weakness of the hind limb. Clinically, in 1805, he ligated an aneurysmal carotid artery, the second time that procedure had been performed. In 1805 Cooper carried out his first carotid ligation followed by long-term survival; the same day he successfully ligated the external iliac artery for a large femoral aneurysm. On nine occasions Cooper performed this procedure using the extraperitoneal approach that bears his name; eight of these patients were long-term survivors. However, his most famous vascular procedure took place at Guy's Hospital on June 25 (26), 1817, when he performed transperitoneal ligation of the abdominal aorta for bleeding aneurysm in the groin. The patient died 40 hours later. Somewhat ironically, in 1820, his baronetcy was the consequence of a minor procedure, the incision and drainage of an infected sebaceous cyst on King George IV.

The essence of Sir Astley Cooper's approach to medical knowledge is expressed in his *Surgical Essays,* "Collecting of evidence upon any medical subject, there are but three sources from which we can hope to obtain it: viz. from observation of the living subject; from examination of the dead; and from experiment on living animals." Feelings regarding the demeanor of a surgeon appear in his *Lectures on Surgery:* "It is the surgeon's duty to tranquilize the temper, to beget cheerfulness, and to impart confidence of recovery."

Landmarks and Ligatures

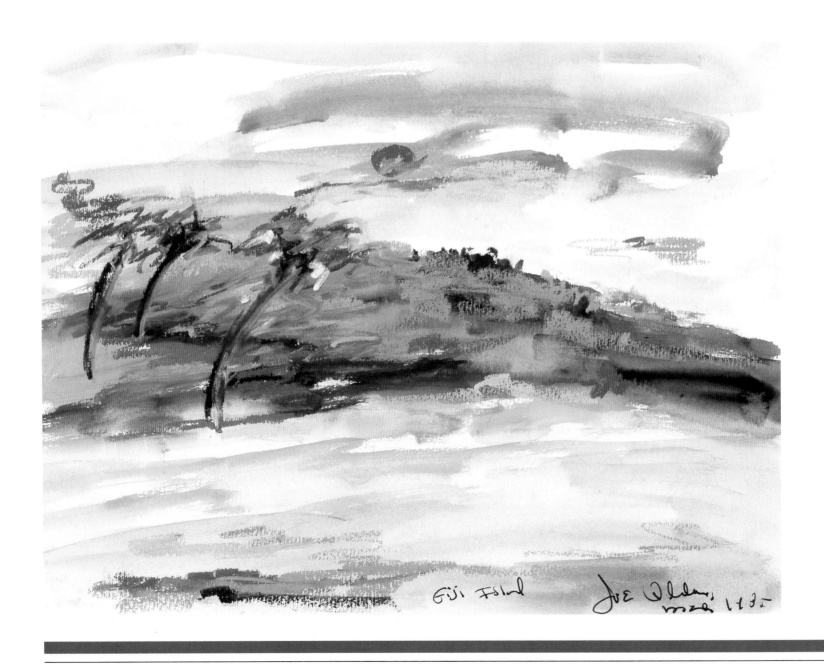

Fiji Islands. 1985. Watercolor, 9 x 12″.

On the fourteenth day of March, 1879, in Ulm, Germany, a lion was born. It was he who said, "Perfection of means and confusion of goals seem to characterize our age." In a prologue to a book entitled, *Where Is Science Going?* he opined, "Many men devote themselves to science . . . because it offers them an opportunity to display their particular talents . . . as an athlete who exhalts in the exercise of his muscular powers. Another class of men come in the hope of securing a profitable return. . . . One of the strongest motives is the urge to flee from daily life with its drab and deadly dullness."

On the twenty-second day of March, in Weimar, Germany, in 1832, a lion uttered his dying words: "Let the light enter." This literary genius, although a law student, was more often found in medical classrooms, because he felt that the art of healing was a portal to understanding nature. This poet devoted a segment of his life to the discovery of a vestigial premaxillary bone in humans because he knew the bone existed in other levels of the animal kingdom. His thesis of "morphology" was based on the concept of unity through diversity, and that man was in conformity with the rest of nature.

One of the major characters in the works of this novelist was an apprentice surgeon, Wilhelm Meister, and it was the author who said that medical students must develop a sense of reverence that takes three forms: what is above him, around him, and beneath him. The greatest of German authors stated, "The physician must be productive if he really intends to heal; if he is not so, he will succeed now and then, as if by chance." Another of his statements relating to research unfortunately still pertains in isolated examples. He wrote, "Thus I saw that most men only care for science so far as they get a living by it, and that they worship even error when it affords them a subsistence." The author who provided us with the most memorable character in German literature, also a physician, had an everlasting regard for medicine and its arena. A multilingual genius, he capsuled his regard for the world of medicine with the statement, "I have learned much from the disease which life could have never taught me anywhere else."

The lion who came in in March was Albert Einstein; the lion who went out in March was the author of *Dr. Faustus*, Johann Wolfgang von Goethe.

A Lion In, A Lion Out

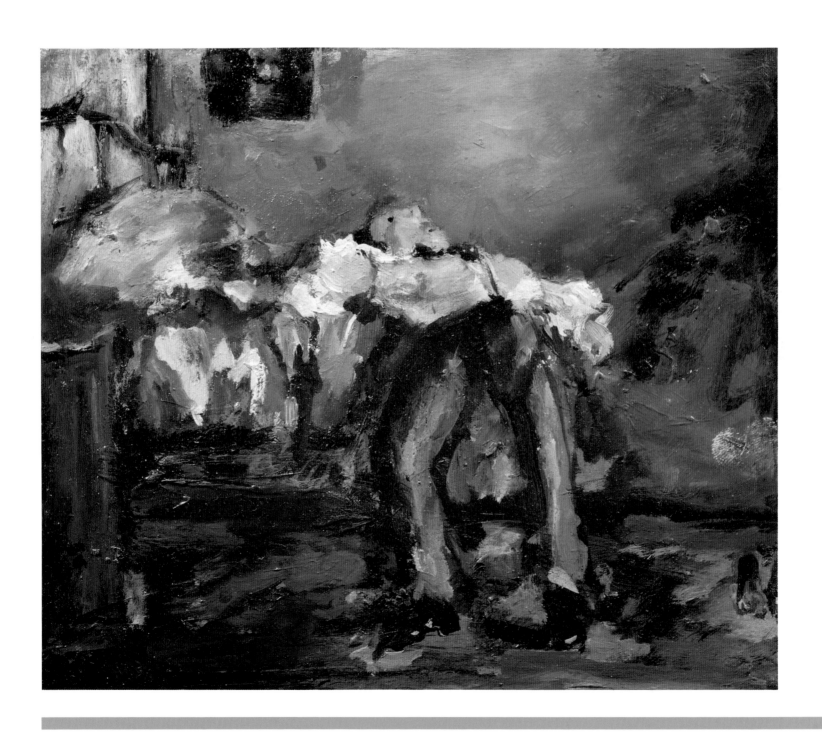

Death of an Artist, after Manet. 1990. Oil on panel, 12 x 10″. Collection Allan Stone.

On December 15, 1837 the life of the man generally regarded as the Father of American Surgery came to an end. It is customary to commemorate a birthdate, but because Philip Syng Physick focused on his death, noting the date of his death is a reasonable alternative. Our distinguished surgical progenitor not only took extreme caution to prevent being buried alive, but also insisted his grave be guarded for 6 weeks so that his body would not be stolen for anatomic dissection, an unusual stance for a surgical anatomist.

Physick was born July 7, 1768 and was persuaded by his father, who had been Keeper of the Great Seal of the Colony of Pennsylvania, to become a surgeon rather than a goldsmith. Following an apprenticeship in Philadelphia, Physick exposed himself to the greatest possible preparation by serving as a favored pupil of John Hunter and then completing studies for a medical degree at Edinburgh.

The designation Father of American Surgery is based on his important contributions as well as the position he held. Initiation of the use of a gastric tube for lavage, invention of a needle forceps to permit ligation of deep vessels, introduction of absorbable (animal) sutures, successful ligation of an arteriovenous aneurysm in 1804, innovations in traction and manipulation for fracture, and stimulation of growth of ununited fracture by the use of a seton are among his notable contributions to the field of surgery. His successful lithotomy of Chief Justice John Marshall bespeaks his clinical eminence. His appointment as professor of surgery at the University of Pennsylvania completes a triple threat with expertise in clinical research, clinical practice, and education. His one apparent major flaw was his reluctance to publish. Throughout his entire career he contributed only six papers, making a total of fewer than 40 pages.

Concerning the issue of fatherhood of our discipline, a devotee of history would refer to the statement by Sir William Osler: "As a teacher you can never get oriented without a knowledge of the Fathers, ancient and modern." But there is also room for the cynicism of historian Henry E. Sigerist, who wrote, "The very popular hunting for fathers of every branch of medicine is foolish; it is unfair not only to mothers and ancestors but to obstetricians and midwives."

Commemorating a Death

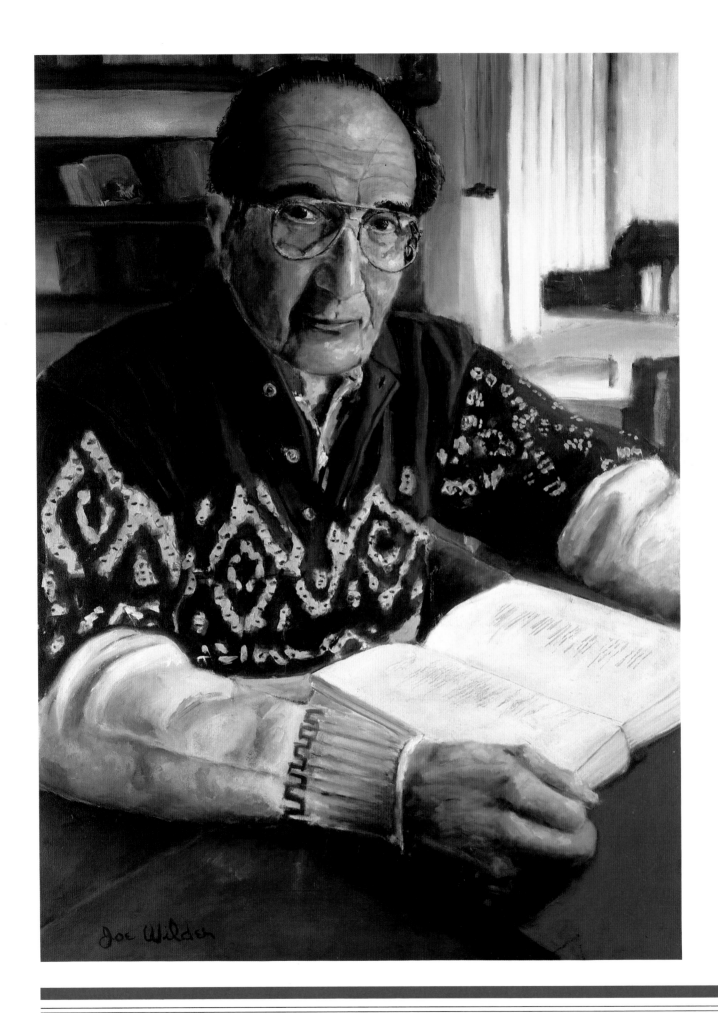

Dr. Salvador E. Luria, Nobel Laureate. 1984. Oil on canvas, 40 x 30″. Collection Massachusetts Institute of Technology.

In 1821, a 25-year-old poet who had initially studied for a medical career lamentably died at the beginning of a brilliant literary career. In the entries of the books kept in the medical offices at Guy's Hospital in London there is a notation that John Keats entered as one of the Physicians' and Surgeons' Pupils and Dressers on October 1, 1815. By July of 1816 he had been examined by the Court and awarded a certificate qualifying him as a practitioner. But John Keats is only one of many medical personalities whose lives were affected by the study of surgery and who made major contributions to our literary heritage.

Thomas Linacre was the founder and first President of the Royal College of Surgeons, yet he was perhaps best known as a scholar of Greek and Latin. Tobias Smollett served as a Surgeon's Mate in the Navy; he is considered the pioneer of the modern novel. Oliver Goldsmith failed his examination at the College of Surgeons and was turned down as a surgeon for the Royal Navy; his contributions of *The Vicar of Wakefield, She Stoops To Conquer,* and *The Deserted Village* led to an honorary degree of Bachelor of Medicine. On the continent the incomparable Ambroise Paré wrote and published sonnets and short verse. Eugene Sue, another French army surgeon, is better known as the author of *The Wandering Jew,* and Johann Christoph Friedrich von Schiller left his career as assistant regimental surgeon to write *Wilhelm Tell.*

A list of American surgeons who have contributed to the pride of our profession must include George David Stewart, a president of the American College of Surgeons and a man regarded as an excellent poet; John Chalmers DaCosta's book was a classic in surgery, and he also published poetry in the classic fashion; Harvey Cushing won the Pulitzer Prize for his biography of Sir William Osler.

The list of physicians who have been part of the literary world does not end with surgeons; an enumeration of nonsurgical medical personalities is truly expansive and would include such names as Luke, Rabelais, Chekhov, Ibsen, and Holmes. Thus, members of our profession who may be regarded as truants by their medical confreres have triumphantly enriched our culture and our society.

Triumphant Truants

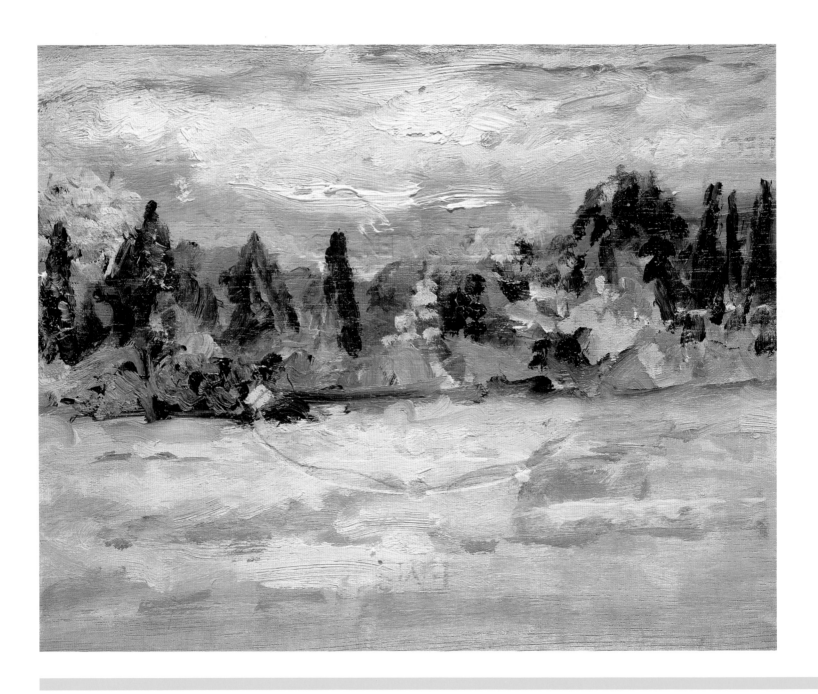

Nature. 1992. Oil on panel, 6 x 8″.

Rudolph Virchow introduced the word "thrombosis." He demonstrated that thrombi in the lungs were part of thrombi from veins of the lower extremities and pelvis and that they were transported by the bloodstream; it was he who named the new pathologic phenomenon "embolism." His major medical contribution was the introduction of the concept of cellular pathology.

A second dimension of this triple-threat man was in anthropology. He was an archaeologist who excavated with Schliemann at the site of Troy, and was also a noted ethnologist and anthropologist. Virchow was credited with the organization of German anthropology. That his authority in German anthropology was considered far greater than that in medicine was a point that greatly disturbed him.

It is the third facet of his accomplishments that merits emphasis—Virchow the statesman. Rudolph Virchow was a member of the Prussian parliament from 1861 to 1902 and a staunch proponent of equal rights for all citizens, aiming for a maximum of self-government. He wrote, "We want that the poor should enjoy on earth a happier life. When people are educated and free everybody will understand and will be able to obtain what he needs. . . ." Virchow was a major opponent of Bismarck and spoke out loudly against anti-Catholic laws and against anti-Semitism.

Although his contributions did much to further the natural scientific elements of modern medicine, Virchow thought that medicine was the most important of the humanistic sciences capable of comprehending mankind, life, and disease, rather than a technical craft. He was a humanist who believed that humanism should be based on natural science and that it stemmed from the individual; he recognized the rights of every individual to develop. He stated that "physicians are the natural attorneys of the poor and social problems should largely be solved by them."

I join him in championing the concept that physicians and surgeons should be counted among the elder statesmen who support the social structure of society, and that there is no other group better suited to propose laws as the basis of social structure. Men and women who are concerned with the science of the healthy and the sick are eminently equipped to address the problems of a healthy or sick society and should replace lawyers, politicians, and financiers in leadership roles.

From Clots to Crypts to Corridors of Decisions

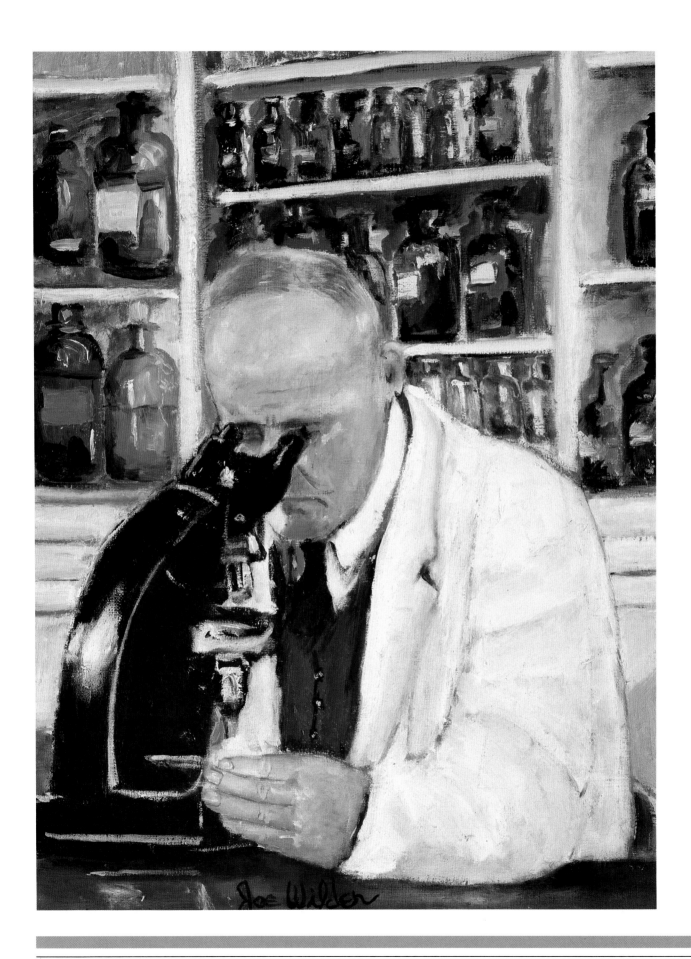

Domagk, Nobel Prize Winner. 1987. Oil on canvas, 12 x 10″.

More than 125 years have passed since the curtain rose on the era of antiseptic surgery. The word "sepsis" is actually a Greek term for putrefaction. Lord Joseph Lister, following the lead of Pasteur, emphasized that putrefaction could not occur in the absence of living organisms.

Lord Lister waited 2 years, until 1867, to publish his first 11 cases demonstrating the success of his method. Although the first application of carbolic acid in March of 1865 failed, Lister persisted. His initial report of the first monumental case reads:

> James G.—aged 11. Admitted on the 12th of August 1865 to Glasgow Royal Infirmary with a compound fracture of the left leg. The house surgeon, Dr. MacFee, acting under instruction, laid a piece of lint dipped in liquid carbolic acid upon the wound and applied lateral pasteboard splints that were left undisturbed for four days. When the wound was examined, there was no suppuration. This no doubt was a favorable case and might have done well under ordinary treatment. But remarkable retardation of suppuration was encouraging.

Lister's work, initially warmly received, was treated then by apathy and antagonism in England, but eventually his contribution was regarded as one of the keystones of modern surgery. Lister the physician wrote, "It is our proud office to tend the fleshy tabernacle of the immortal spirit, and our path, if rightly followed, will be guided by unfettered truth and love unfeigned." Lister the surgeon said, "To intrude an unskilled hand into such a piece of divine mechanism as the human body is indeed a fearful responsibility." Lister the educator stated, "You must always be students, learning and unlearning to your life's end, and if, gentlemen, you are not prepared to follow your profession in this spirit, I implore you to leave its ranks and take yourself to some third-class trade."

Lister's role in surgery is almost unparalleled. Sir Berkeley Moynihan indicated that "on the role of honor which, in letters of gold, bears the name of the saviours of mankind, no man is more worthy of remembrance than Lister." But how has his name been perpetuated? In the *Oxford English Dictionary* there are four listings specifically based on his name: "listerism" refers to the system of surgery originated by him; "listerian" is the adjective, and "listerize," to treat according to Lister's principle. These three terms have atrophied from disuse, leaving only Listerine, an antiseptic solution (although not truly antiseptic) used as a mouthwash. The trademark is recognized by all. How many appreciate the origin of the name?

Lister's Legacy

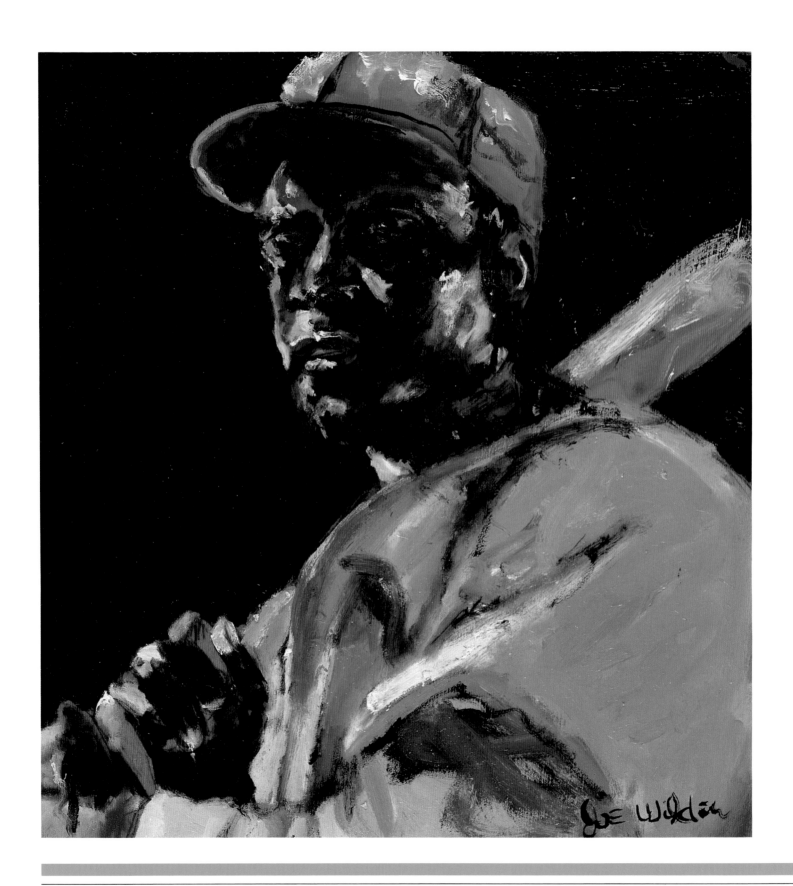

Jackie Robinson. 1987. Oil on panel. 12 x 12″. Collection Nick Wilder.

On January 6, the Baker Street Irregulars celebrate the birthday of Sherlock Holmes. A lean, wiry man with an aquiline nose and piercing eyes that took in everything, sizing up his man in a moment. A clearcut mouth and beautiful strong, supple, dextrous hands; the possessor of the precise high-pitched voice that said, "Gentlemen, I am not quite sure whether this man is a corkcutter or a slater. I observe a slight callus or hardening on the outside of his thumb." The description, the man, and the words are not those of the great detective but rather those of the Edinburgh surgeon who taught Arthur Conan Doyle and who became the prototype for his central character.

I find it gratifying that it was a surgeon's diagnostic acumen that made such a vivid impression on a young medical student who then modeled the extraordinary Sherlock Holmes after the surgeon. The role model for Sherlock Holmes was a Mr. Joseph Bell (1837-1911). From 1771 through 1911, without a break, either a Benjamin or a Joseph Bell was on the roll of the Royal College of Surgeons. Great-grandfather Benjamin, grandfather Joseph, and father Benjamin (himself a president), preceded *the* Joseph Bell, who served as President from 1887 to 1889. A special assistant to Professor Syme, Joseph Bell attained the post of Senior Surgeon at the Royal Infirmary.

As Professor Caird wrote in Bell's obituary, "Bell was an excellent operator, dextrous, rapid and neat. . . . His diagnostic acumen, his keen powers of observation, his skill in eliciting facts, his sense of humour, enlivened many a charming clinic, and sent his delighted hearers away conscious that their time had been well spent, and that they indeed learned much from an able surgeon who was apt to teach, tactful, impressive, and of ripe experience."

The surgical role model for a fictional character might also function in the same capacity for all modern surgical educators who would ascribe to his epitaph, "Brief, lucid, almost epigrammatic in the use of his words, equally smart and efficient with his knife."

Role Model

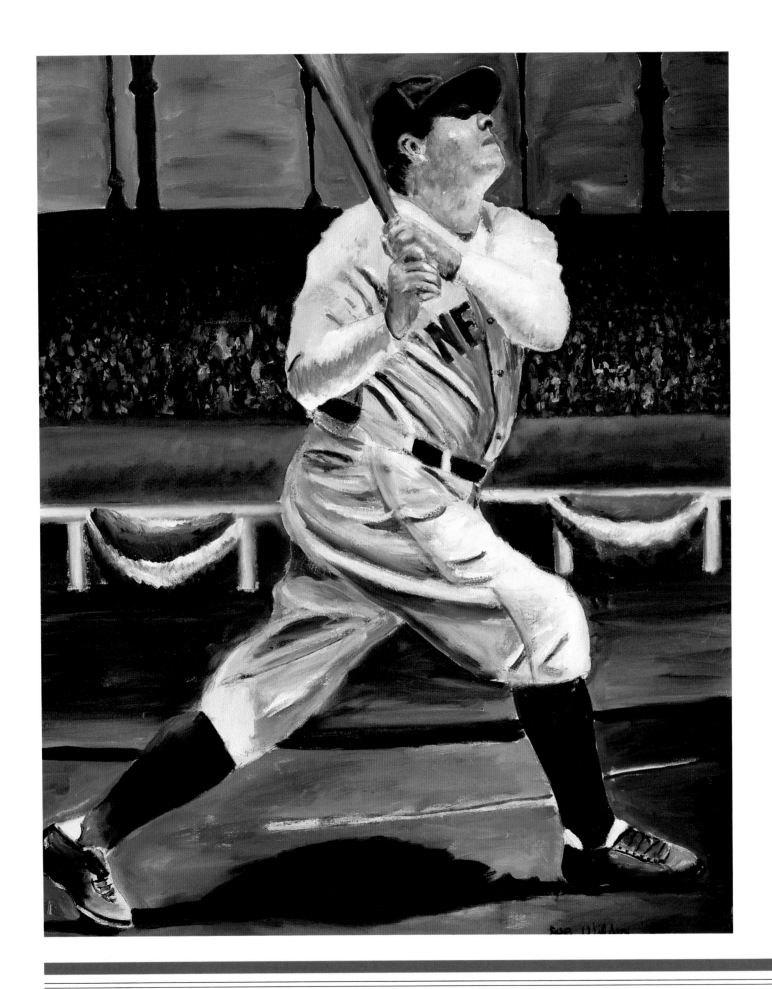

Babe Ruth. 1984. Oil on canvas, 30 x 24″. Collection Cynthia Wilder.

What American surgeon has had the greatest impact on the current science and practice of surgery and medicine in general? What surgeon, whose contributions to the surgical literature consisted of only a graduate thesis on the surgical treatment of epilepsy and an extensive review of the history and literature of surgery from 1552 B.C. to A.D. 1894, could have been so important? Who was it who began his career as a military surgeon, documented no significant operation, never held a surgical professorship, yet still merits heroic status?

The subject in question was medical director of the Army of the Potomac, overseeing the practice of surgery, and then worked as assistant surgeon general. In that venue he dedicated his work to increasing the size of the library and to cataloguing all medical literature. In 1879, he brought out the first of the monthly *Index Medicus;* in 1880, he published the first of 14 volumes of the *Index Catalogue.*

About medical literature, he wrote, "There is a vast amount of this effete and worthless material in the literature of medicine . . . which has been characterized as 'superlatively middling, the quintessential extract of mediocrity.' Nine-tenths, at least, of it becomes worthless, and of no interest within ten years after the date of its publication, and much of it so when it first appears."

Another sphere of influence was in hospital design. It was he who sketched the plans for the Johns Hopkins Hospital and influenced the design of, and conduct within, hospitals throughout the world. His thesis is evidenced in his statement, "A sick man enters the hospital to have his pain relieved—his disease cured. To the end the mental influences brought to bear upon him are always important, sometimes more so than the physical . . . he is not to have his feelings hurt by being, against his will, brought before a large class of unsympathetic noisy students."

A pioneer in preventive medicine and vital statistics, for a brief period the director of the hospital of the University of Pennsylvania, he devoted the last 17 years of his life to the nonmedical arena of literature at the New York Public Library, where he consolidated the collections of the Astor, Lenox, and Tilden foundations into a single library, designed the building on 42nd Street, and blueprinted a city-wide satellite library system.

One man's efforts contribute on a daily basis to our learning process as we seek a citation in the library, and on a daily basis to our patient practice as we make rounds in our modern hospitals. That man of extraordinary influence was John Shaw Billings.

A Man of Extraordinary Influence

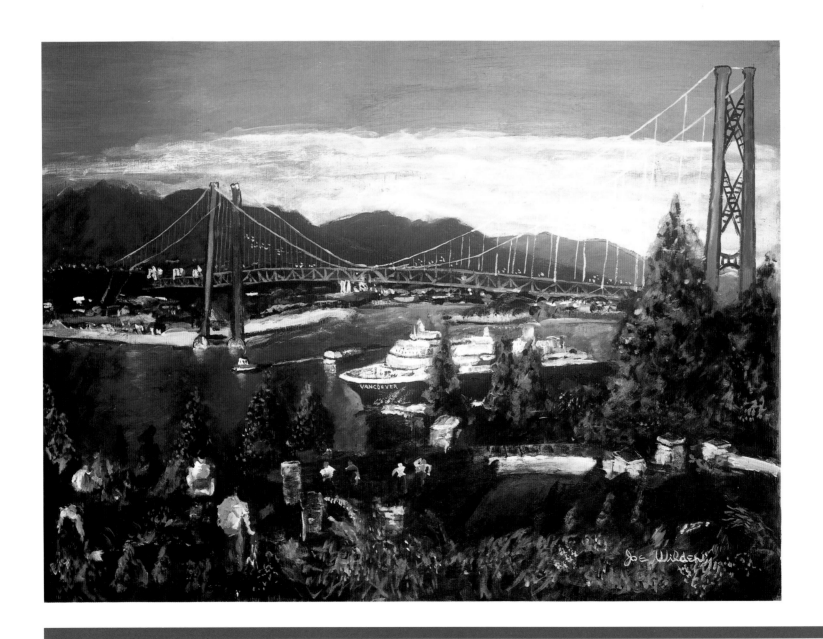

Vancouver. 1989. Oil on canvas, 12 x 18″. Collection Roerig, a division of Pfizer Pharmaceuticals.

The most publicized drainage of an appendiceal abscess was performed in Buckingham Palace. On June 24, 1902, Edward VII, with a 10-day history of appendicitis and a distinct mass in the right lower quadrant, insisted on going to Westminster Abbey for the coronation, to which his distinguished surgeon, Sir Frederick Treves, replied, "Then, Sir, you'll go as a corpse." The King agreed to submit to an operation just 48 hours before the coronation, at which time an appendiceal abscess was drained, with no mention made of the removal of the appendix. On August 9, just 7 weeks after the procedure, the coronation ceremony took place.

The responsible surgeon had been a teacher of anatomy who demonstrated a "clear and incisive style and a genius for the telling and humorous phrase." The author of the 1883 Royal College of Surgeons' Jacksonian prize essay performed his first operation on the appendix in 1887, correcting an appendicular distortion without excision of the organ—certainly not a very auspicious beginning. Thereafter, Treves advised treatment of selected cases of "relapsing perityphlitis" by deliberate removal of the appendix during a quiescent period. Ironically, his own daughter died as a consequence of perforation before the surgeon's knife could save her.

The most successful English surgeon of his time, Treves retired at the age of 55 to devote himself to travel and to chronicling his journeys. The panorama of his publications includes highly regarded medical books: *Acute Peritonitis, Anatomy of the Intestinal Canal and Peritoneum, A Manual of Operative Surgery, The Student's Handbook of Surgical Operations, Surgical Applied Anatomy, Scrofula and its Gland Diseases,* and *A Manual of Surgery.* His books on travel at home and abroad remain classics in English literature and include such titles as *Highways and Byways of Dorset, The Other Side of the Lantern, The Cradle of the Deep; An Account of a Voyage to The West Indies,* and *The Land That Is Desolate; An Account of a Tour in Palestine.*

But the bridge from Buckingham to Broadway is related to another of his works. This chronicled Treves' protective care of John Thomas Merrick, who had "the figure of a man with the characteristics of an elephant." In 1923, the year of Treves' death at age 70, he published *The Elephant Man and Other Reminiscences,* consisting of stories of his early days at the London Hospital. It is this work that served as the basis for the Tony Award–winning Broadway drama, *The Elephant Man.*

Buckingham to Broadway

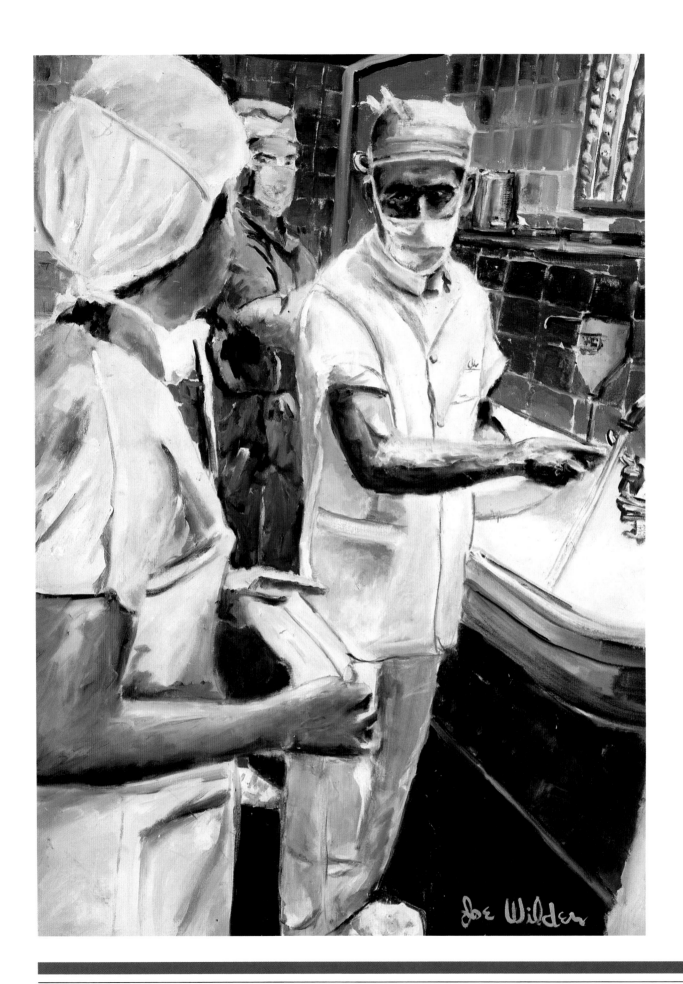

Scrubbing Hands. 1987. Oil on canvas, 30 x 22″.

Should a brief consideration of the contributions of William Stewart Halsted (1852-1922) dwell on the earliest of his meaningful contributions? As a newly appointed 25-year-old house physician at New York Hospital, Halsted designed a temperature, pulse, and respiration chart that remained in use in several hospitals for more than 100 years. Should I interject a note of the personal courage and pioneering spirit of a man who successfully transfused his hemorrhaging sister with his own blood in 1881? Or should I devote the space to his classic clinical contributions: hernia repair, radical mastectomy, and vascular surgery, including the first excision of a subclavian artery aneurysm in 1891?

I could emphasize the scientific aspect and recall that Halsted introduced conduction anesthesia, demonstrated that the submucosa of the intestine provided the strength in an anastomosis, reported successful autografting of a parathyroid gland (the subsequent removal of which caused tetany), and showed that a reimplanted limb could be sustained solely by a collateral blood supply.

Or I could focus on the domain of the general surgeon—the biliary tract—and provide a mix of science and drama. In 1882, Halsted traveled to his mother's home in Albany, where he incised her gallbladder, which was distended with pus, and extracted seven stones. His mother lived for 2 years after what was probably Halsted's first operation on the gallbladder. In 1893, he performed the first three choledochotomies in the United States. In 1896, he successfully carried out the first excision of a carcinoma of the ampulla of Vater, transplanting the common duct into the duodenum. In 1915, cognizant of the significance of a prolonged biliary fistula as a cause of loss of appetite and extreme lethargy, he devised a method of closing an incision in the common duct, which was then drained via a tube coursing through the cystic duct. Ironically, in 1919 Halsted underwent cholecystectomy and removal of a calculus from his common duct, but his technique could not be applied because of the anomalous location of his cystic duct and he suffered for 3 weeks from the consequences of an almost complete bile

Ashes Rest in Brooklyn; the Flame Burns On

leak. In 1922, he was reoperated for recurrent cholangitis and had extraction of a common duct stone. He died postoperatively of pneumonia, and his ashes were laid to rest in Brooklyn cemetery.

But in every practicing surgeon there is a glow of the incandescence from the concepts that arose, particularly at the Johns Hopkins Hospital, under Halsted's stewardship. Rene Leriche referred to Halsted's domain as "the cradle of contemporary surgery." Succeeding generations of American surgeons continue to reflect his luminescence, adhering to his dictum that a surgeon should respect not only the life of the individual but also that of the tissues of the individual and should endeavor not to interfere with the body's natural defense.

As an avowed worshipper of heroes and the past, I continually remind myself of Halsted's enunciation of the adverse position: "It is now, as it was then and as it may ever be; conceptions from the past blind us to facts which almost slap us in the face."

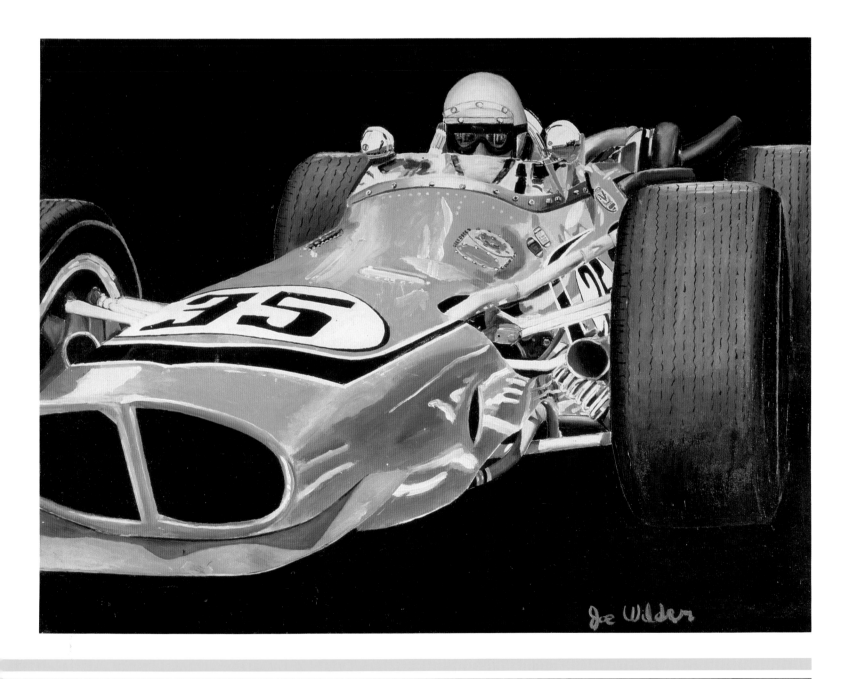

97   *No. 35 at Indy.* 1972. Oil on canvas, 38 x 47".

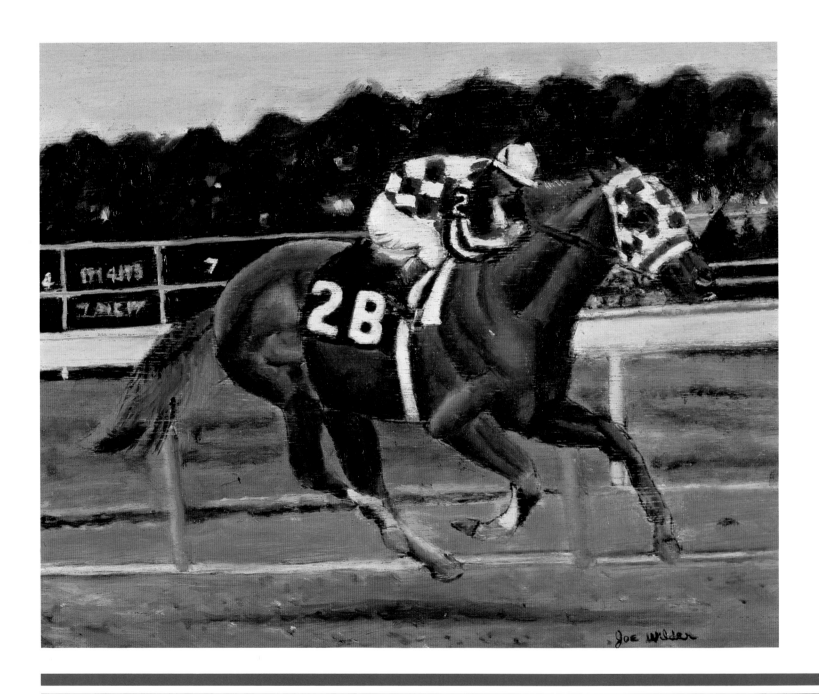

Secretariat, Setting World Record at Belmont, Sept. 15, 1973.
1986. Oil on panel, 11 x 14″. Collection Philip Morris Companies, Inc.

In 1869, the ninth child of a third-generation physician was born in Cleveland. The child, Harvey Cushing, was to become the leading neurologic surgeon in the world by combining his knowledge of fundamental neurophysiology and neuropathology with an inventive surgical technique. He may be described as a Renaissance man because of his activities as a bibliophile and collector who founded the Yale Library of Medical History and as a literary figure whose most highly acclaimed work was a definitive biography of Sir William Osler.

Benjamin Disraeli wrote, "We all of us live too much in a circle." No medical giant's life better conforms to this geometric figure than that of Harvey Cushing. From his place of birth on the Western Reserve of Ohio, he traveled to Yale for his undergraduate education and proceeded to medical school at Harvard, followed by residency training at Johns Hopkins. His role as a surgeon, educator, and literary contributor began at Johns Hopkins, was translocated to Harvard, and ended at Yale. He died at New Haven, and the final arc of the circle was completed when his ashes joined those of his parents in Ohio.

I am reminded of mime Marcel Marceau's interpretation of Shakespeare's famous speech, "All the world's a stage," in *As You Like It,* where the cycle of the seven stages of man are poetically defined. In the pantomime, the beginning is depicted as the fetal position and a return to that position signifies the end.

Although the cycle to death is inevitable, as a romantic I believed that there was an immortality that should be possible for the names of those who contributed significantly—and then a vignette came to mind.

A few years ago, I was giving the American Board of Surgery oral certifying examination to a candidate who dazzled my co-examiner and me with his fund of knowledge and his unassailable approaches to the posed clinical problems. As he was exiting from a perfect exposition, my co-examiner asked, "By the way, who was Harvey Cushing?" Our unqualified enthusiasm was dampened by the answer, "His name doesn't ring a bell, but I think he was a famous English physiologist."

So even the name that is bestowed may be returned to obscurity. There is truth in the line from Emily Dickinson's poem, "Fame is a fickle food upon a shifting plate."

The Name Has a Ring

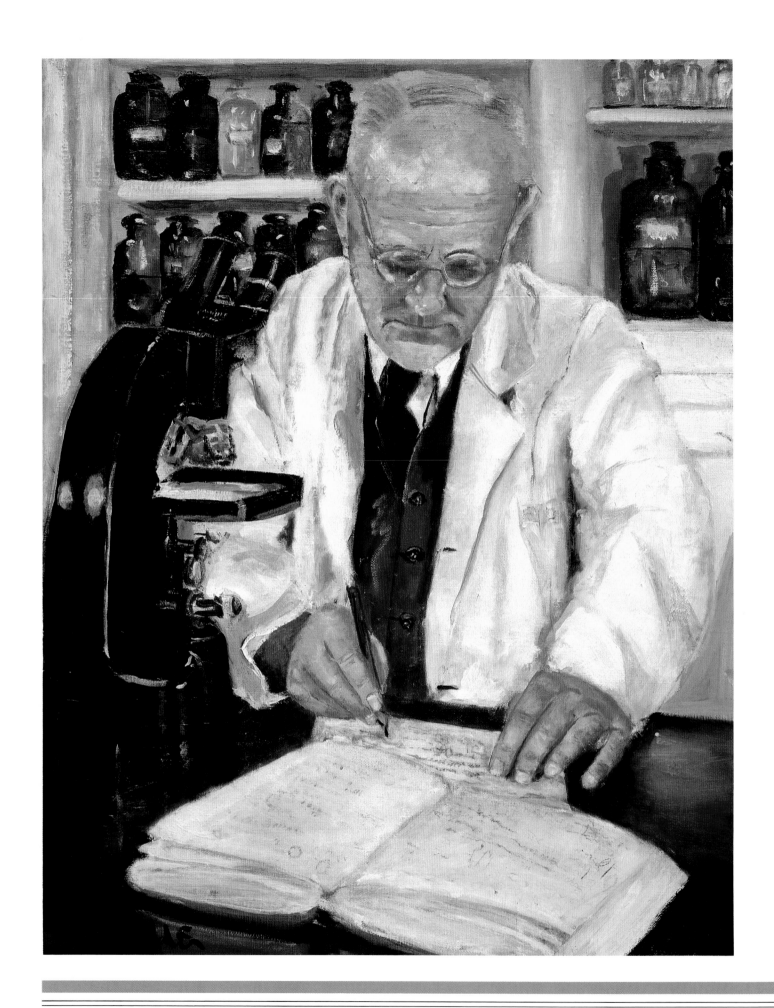

Domagk, Nobel Prize Winner, Making Notes. 1987. Oil on canvas, 24 x 24″.

Were I to ask savant senior surgeons, "Who was Keynes?" I'm quite sure the majority would identify a famous economist who has given his name to the "Keynesian" theory of economics. This response overlooks the economist's younger brother, Geoffrey, one of the most distinguished surgeons of the twentieth century, born in 1887.

In 1981, Geoffrey Keynes published an autobiography entitled *The Gates of Memory*, chronicling 94 years of a remarkable life serving surgery and literature during what, in his own words, was "a quite outrageously enjoyable existence." As a literary personality he published biographies of many English authors. His biography of William Blake and his three-volume edition of Blake's writings rekindled interest in that mystic poet-artist.

As a distinguished surgeon, three contributions stand out: He organized the first transfusion service in London at St. Bartholomew's Hospital (Bart's) after World War I. In 1922, he began experimenting with local radiation of breast cancer. From 1929 on, he was publicly advocating conservative treatment for cancer of the breast. He was recognized as the first champion of what has become an acceptable therapeutic regimen, and in consequence, George Crile dedicated his 1967 book on the subject "To Sir Geoffrey Keynes, whose wisdom and foresight made him the first to resist the trend toward ever more radical treatment of breast cancer."

Following a 1939 report by Alfred Blalock, Keynes began extensive and ongoing work with thymectomy for myasthenia gravis; at one time he had the largest personal experience with this procedure in the world. In his autobiography, there are several memorable statements: In reference to the dogma espousing radical operation for carcinoma of the breast, he wrote, "Every patient had become a 'case,' not an individual, whereas in fact there was good reason for regarding each patient as a separate problem for careful consideration according to individual circumstances. I have ever since that time tried to eliminate the word 'case' from the writings. It had become a universal curse to medical thinking and still is."

As one who has spent a lifetime in a medical academic career, I appreciate that the reasoning which led Keynes to enter private practice focuses on several important and meritorious points: ". . . I had decided not to attempt this [academic career], the main

Recommended Reading

consideration being that the practice of surgery was the central passion of my life. I was a craftsman by instinct, not a teacher, an administrator, a committee man, or a medical politician, as I had noticed that the Professor had to be. I did not dislike teaching and enjoyed the company of students but I had many outside interests. . . . In addition, I had a growing family of sons who had to be educated. All these things required a larger income than was awarded to a Professor, and could only be provided by private practice; this had the additional advantage of fulfilling my desire to have human relations with a proportion of my patients, which one loses if they are all confined in hospital beds as 'cases'."

Perhaps the most succinct and poignant expression of factors that may contribute to the choice of surgery as a career came from the pen of this 94-year-old distinguished retiree. "I was sorry for the physicians. They had hard intellectual work judging the patient's personality and arriving at a diagnosis by observation of signs and symptoms, but, that done, there were but few really specific drugs and the 'doctor' could only try to create the best circumstance in which the natural processes could enable the patient to cure himself; whereas a surgeon having diagnosed, proceeded to cure the patient by the skill of his own hands, a much more positive satisfaction for the medical man. A surgeon is a craftsman, basing his craft on a wide knowledge of structure and biology, always gaining by experience of the results of his work."

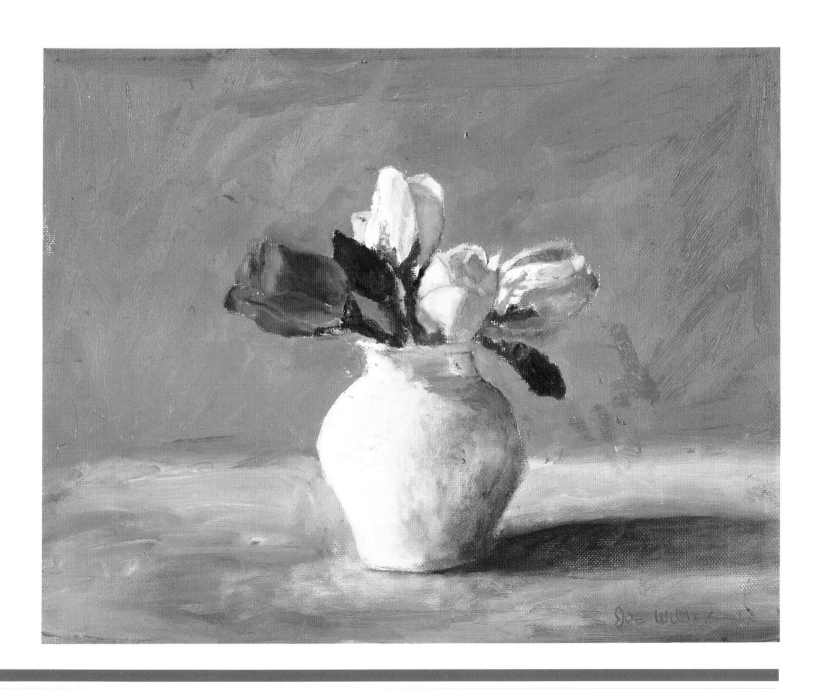

103   *Four Roses*. 1986. Oil on canvas, 11 x 14″. Collection Mr. and Mrs. Bruce Verstandig.

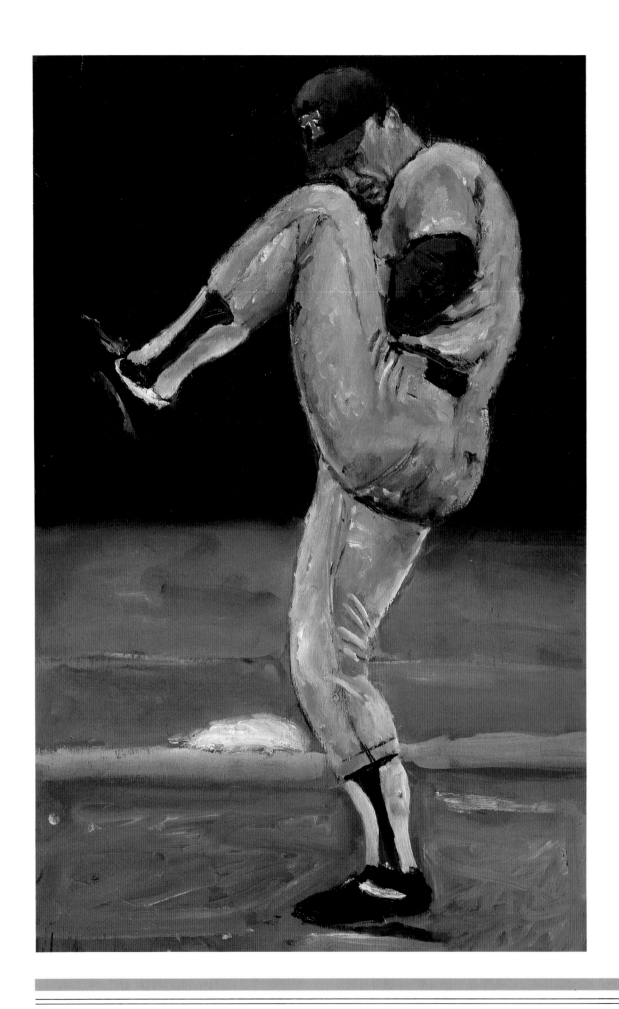

Nolan Ryan. 1991. Oil on panel, 18 x 12″.

Consideration of a list of medical Nobel Laureates provides the editorial prerogative of satisfying a vicarious desire—that of contributing to the selection of the prize winners and of righting wrongs. It is relatively easy to find room for another name; we merely have to scratch two prizes given for clinical accomplishments that have had no lasting or meaningful applicability. How many patients have benefitted by malarial inoculation for the treatment of dementia paralytica of central nervous system syphilis (the 1972 prize)? Although Egas Moniz aided mankind by the introduction of his pioneer work in arteriography, the contribution for which he won the 1949 prize was the discovery of the therapeutic value or prefrontal leukotomy in certain psychoses. Has this procedure stood the test of time?

On the other hand, there was a surgical contribution that went unrecognized by the committee in Stockholm, a contribution that has formed the basis of an entire discipline and a modern industry. In 1938 John H. Gibbon, Jr., reported his success with an extracorporeal pump oxygenator in experimental animals. On May 6, 1953, Dr. Gibbon also first successfully applied the pump oxygenator to a clinical situation; it sustained all cardiac function for 26 minutes to permit the repair of a large interatrial septal defect. As Dr. Gibbon humbly stated when he first presented his clinical experience, "It seems to me that there will always be a place for an extracorporeal blood circuit because it permits a longer, safer interval for opening the heart."

According to the specifics enumerated in the will of Alfred Nobel establishing the Prize—"to honor those who during the preceding year have conferred the greatest benefit to mankind"—John H. Gibbon, Jr. certainly qualified. Although Gibbon died prematurely, fortunately he lived to see the burgeoning consequences of his continued efforts and his thoughts might well have been those verbalized by another surgeon whose influence was panoramic. Lord Joseph Lister stated in his address at Edinburgh in 1898:

> I must confess that highly, and very highly, as I esteem the honours which have been conferred upon me, I regard that all worldly distinctions are as nothing in comparison with the hope that I may have been the means of reducing in some degree the sum of human misery.

Strike Two, Add One!

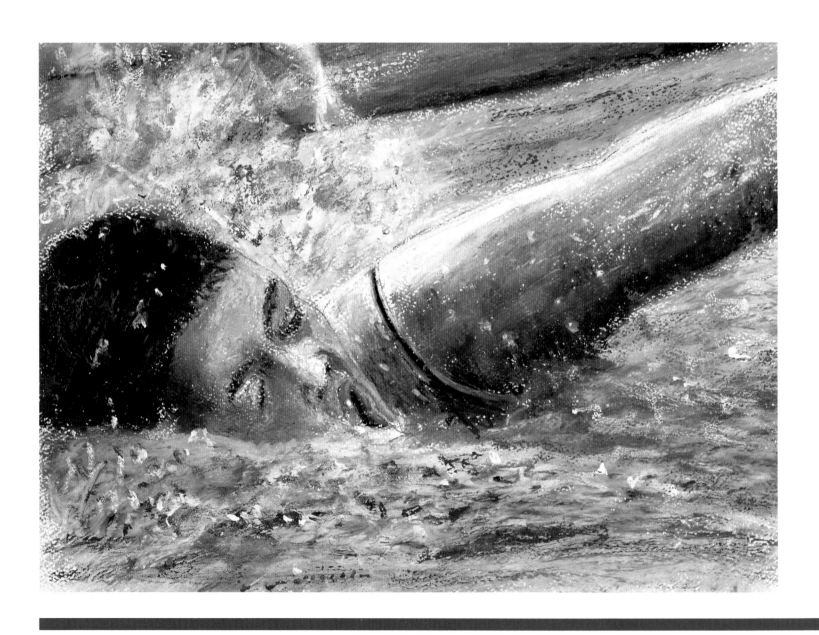

Women's Freestyle Finals, 1980 Olympics. 1984. Watercolor, pastel, and oil on paper, 10 x 14".

*S*everal years ago the United States Postal Service brought out a commemorative stamp honoring Dr. Harvey Cushing. How many physicians have been so honored? How many were surgeons? And what distinguished the recipients who received this honor posthumously?

Eleven stamps have been issued commemorating distinguished physicians. Surgery can claim, with pride, six of these. The first physician so honored was Crawford W. Long, the Georgia surgeon and anesthetist who administered sulfuric ether anesthesia on March 30, 1842, more than 4 years before Morton's administration of it at the Massachusetts General Hospital. Long did not publish until December 1849, by which time he had accumulated eight cases, and so Morton could not have known of the event. In 1940, 1 week after issue of the stamp honoring Crawford Long, a stamp commemorating the activities of Walter Reed appeared. The third physician honored on a stamp was Ephraim McDowell, who in 1809 performed the first celiotomy and ovariotomy. That stamp appeared in 1951. Five years later, the faces of Drs. William James and Charles Horace Mayo appeared on a stamp. In 1968, Oliver Wendell Holmes, Professor of Anatomy and distinguished author, was honored. Six years after this, a stamp commemorating the first female doctor in America was issued. Elizabeth Blackwell was an 1849 graduate of the Geneva Medical School of Western New York and eventually became the Professor of Gynecology at the London School of Medicine for women. In 1978, George Papanicolaou and his Pap smear received the philatelic commemoration. In 1981, one of our most distinguished black surgeons, Charles R. Drew, appeared on a stamp. As a fellow and resident in surgery at Columbia Presbyterian Hospital, Drew worked in the area of fluid, electrolyte, and colloid balance, and he coauthored a paper entitled "The Preservation of Blood," presented at the American Surgical Association in 1942. In 1986, the distinguished cardiologist Paul Dudley White was honored.

The final "surgeon" to be honored before Cushing represents the featured player of an extraordinary story. Dr. Mary Walker, a graduate of the Syracuse Medical School in 1855, served for 3 years in the Civil War as a nurse and an assistant surgeon, perhaps a spy, and received the Medal of Honor, actually bestowed too liberally during that time. Subsequent to the war, she did little in the field of surgery, and it is questionable whether she practiced medicine. In 1917, her name was formally removed from the list of the recipients of the Medal of Honor. In the 1980s, related perhaps to the movement for women's rights, her name was reinstated on the list of those who received the Medal of Honor, and in 1982 this was specifically designated on a commemorative stamp.

There is little question that each of the individuals commemorated on a stamp was distinguished. It would be intriguing to be privy to the deliberation involved in the selection process. One can only wonder at this process, since the one medical field specifically honored on a stamp is osteopathic medicine.

Stamps of Approval

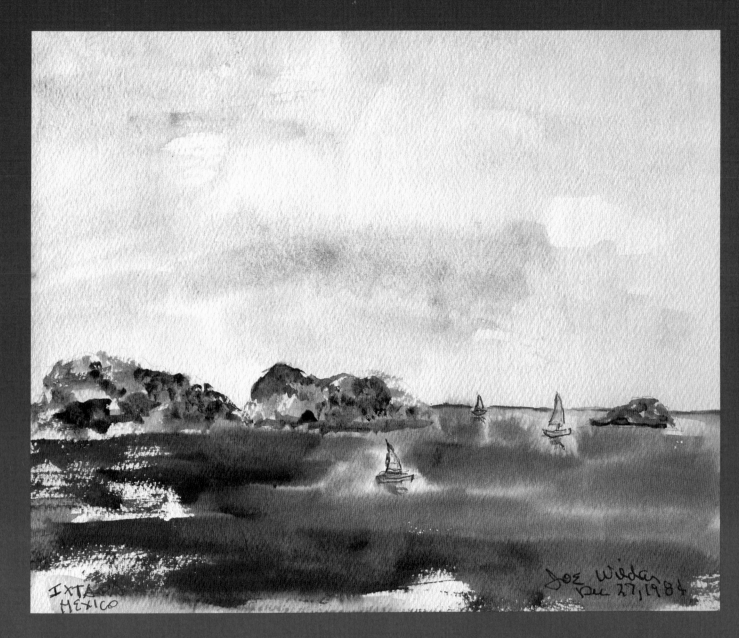

IXTAPA
MEXICO

Joe Wilder
Dec 27, 1988

PART FIVE

Ethics and
Education

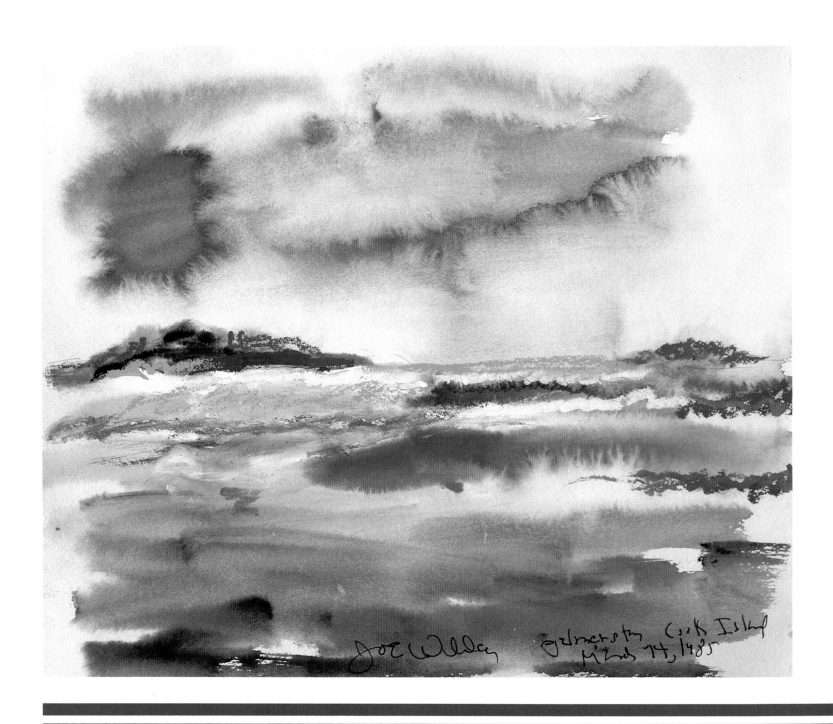

Palmerston, Cook Island, South Pacific. 1985. Watercolor, 9 x 10½″.

Medical ethics is a chameleon, ever changing with the environment. In the lexicon of the Sydenham Society of the 1880s, medical ethics was defined as "the laws of duties of medical men to the public, to each other, and to themselves with regard to the exercise of their profession."

Modern medicine is evolving into a scientific technology as opposed to a humane art. The prevailing perception regards people as if they were machines and disease as an interruption of the machine's efficiency. Technologic advances have been accompanied by concern over genetic alteration, contraception, deliberate interruption of pregnancy, transplantation, and mechanical rebuilding and immortalization. Ask a physician or surgeon why a specific regimen has been adopted and the answer will refer to the opinions of leaders in the field and personal experiences. Ask the same person, however, to defend an ethical consideration related to patient care or medical research and the response will most likely be emotional. Articulations about ethics are usually based on visceral responses—products of familial and perhaps religious influences early in life and impressions gained over the years. The vital element that is absent is a sound intellectual base evolved from an acquaintance with the pertinent facts and literature.

Science is basically concerned with true and false, not good and evil. However, although science is amoral, scientists are not. Throughout history the primary forces behind the development of codes of ethics have been the physicians themselves. Hippocrates proposed what was at the time a radical standard in that his code opposed the prevailing Greek mores of abortion, infanticide, homosexuality, and euthanasia. In 1803, Thomas Percival published his *Medical Ethics*, which served as the progenitor of the code that the AMA formulated at its first meeting in 1847; it has since been revised four times. Ethics for experiments on human subjects were proposed in the Nuremberg Code of 1947 and expressed by the World Medical Association in the Declaration of Helsinki in 1964. The possible scientific basis for ethics is delineated in Julian and Thomas Henry Huxley's *Touchstone for Ethics*, 1893-1943, and C.H. Waddington's *Science and Ethics*.

As Chauncey D. Leake wrote: "The moral problems arising from modern biomedical progress . . . are the responsibility of all intelligent people and will require extensive social consideration before socially acceptable solutions to these problems may be agreed upon." In this age of scientific advancement, we as physicians have increasing influence on our fellow beings. The proper use of this power demands a deliberate assessment of the values on which our systems of ethics are based.

Values do not just exist but are subjectively created. The values that Hippocrates championed are important only in historical perspective. Medical ethics demand the chameleon's characteristic of change, but unlike the colors of the chameleon, which blend into the background, the image of ethical change should be conspicuous.

Evolving Ethics

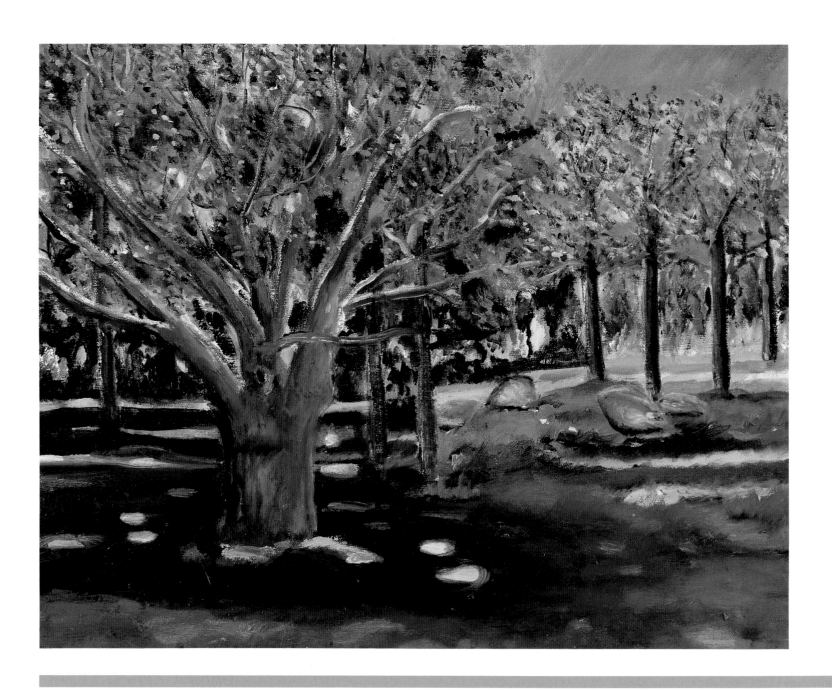

The Great Maple Tree. 1980. Oil on canvas, 14 x 18″.

With increased life expectancy and with the evolution of more sophisticated procedures, particularly in the fields of cardiovascular and orthopedic surgery, operating on octogenarians is a much more common occurrence. It has become more and more appropriate to reflect on old age and the problems of longevity and to consider that old age is in itself a prolonged infirmity. As Antiphanes stated, old age is the sanctuary of ills.

At the age of 58 Thomas Jefferson wrote, "My only fear is that I may live too long." A positive attitude toward aging was expressed in Alfred Lord Tennyson's poem, "Ulysses": "Old age hath yet his honor and his toil; Death closes all: but something in the end, some look of noble note, may yet be done." And as a proverb states, "All would live long, but none would be old." At some time protracted life becomes protracted woe. It is at this point that the physician must help to resolve the ethical problem of granting the patient added days or years, devoid of added living.

In the early seventeenth century Sir Francis Bacon reflected on the field of medicine in *Advancement of Learning* and proposed that "the lengthening of the thread of life itself and the postponement of a time of death, which gradually steals on by natural dissolution and the decay of age, is a subject which no physician has handled in proportion to its dignity." A mere 15 years ago, the great Boston physician James Howard Means similarly declared that he felt young doctors had inadvertently been trained to consider it a virtue to prolong life for the sole purpose of prolonging it.

Surgeons must question whether it is meaningful to the patient to augment flow to one portion of the body, to extend the range of motion of one joint, or to remove an asymptomatic malignancy. The question becomes particularly pertinent when the patient evidences frank senility and is a ward of society.

As we contemplate an operation we can carry off with competence, we, as surgeons and humanists, should balance the equation of indications and contraindications, and reflect on the philosophy expressed in *The Doctor's Dilemma* by Louis Lasagna, "Medicine might consider forsaking the worship of the Goddess Longevity—can the man whose life is not rich really profit from its extension?"

Longevity

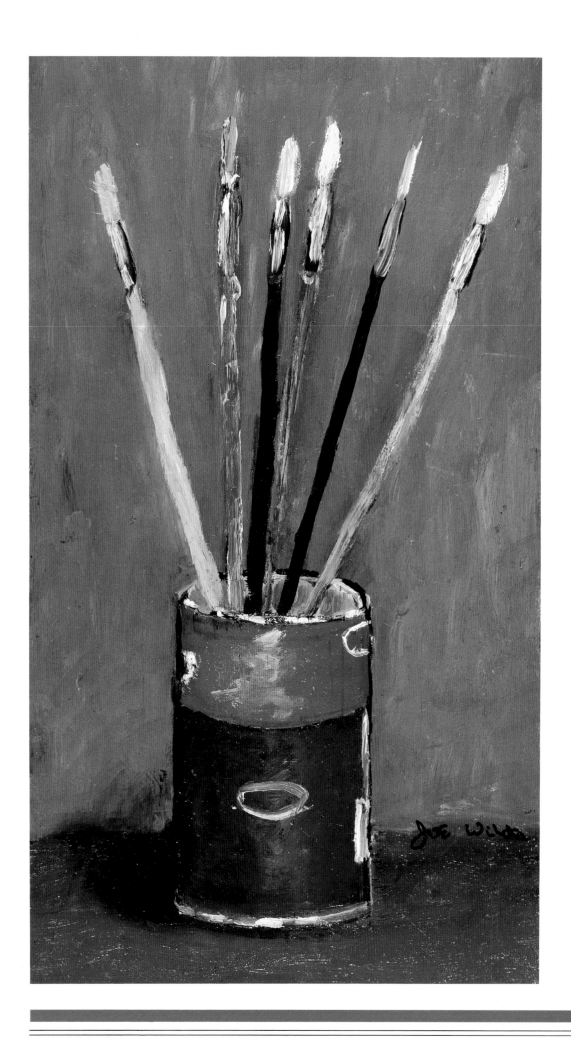

Can of My Brushes. 1981. Oil on panel, 14 x 8″. Collection Joan Wolff.

The medical education committee of our university recently held a retreat. Perhaps the word "retreat" is more appropriate than advance, because we frequently return to old, discarded, and what were, at times, maligned approaches. We gathered to consider the curriculum and the process of imparting knowledge.

The word "Curriculum" often appears with a capital letter, while the word "teacher" is presented in small print. "It is one thing to sit and theorize about teaching, and quite another to find people capable of carrying out our altogether admirable ideas." We frequently structure the *curriculum* based on what the teacher wants to teach rather than what the student should be learning, forgetting that "the measure of a teacher's success lies not in his or her own ideas but in those which radiate from pupils."

A process of progressive decentralization has evolved, and we now teach from independent departmental blocks with little appreciation of what is actually needed for the education of a physician. What surgeon has not been appalled by the third-year student's lack of appreciation of anatomy during a specific procedure in a given operation? "Preclinical chairs are occupied by men whose scientific interests are unrelated to anything that has to do with medicine." Many clinical chairs are occupied by men or women disinterested in patient care, which they regard as anathema.

Surgery makes a unique contribution to education. In a short time a student following surgical patients is exposed to triage, clinical and laboratory evaluations, and reasoning processes in relation to therapy and its results. The study of chronic disease cannot provide as much breadth and depth of experience in as short a time.

I certainly agree with Lord Brain that the curriculum should not be "a honeycomb in which individual bees add cell to cell, but rather a cerebral cortex in which all cells are functionally related." The curriculum for a medical student must be directed at an end point, appreciating that more than 90% of the graduates intend to practice the art and science of medicine, and provisions should be made for developing the *art* aspect. The curriculum committee should be made up of teachers who should exercise their influence nonterritorially, recognizing as Harvey Cushing did that "the best any of us can do as successful teachers of medical students is to instill principles, arouse interest, put the student on the right track, give him methods, show him how to study, and early to discern between essentials and unessentials."

Curriculum Considered

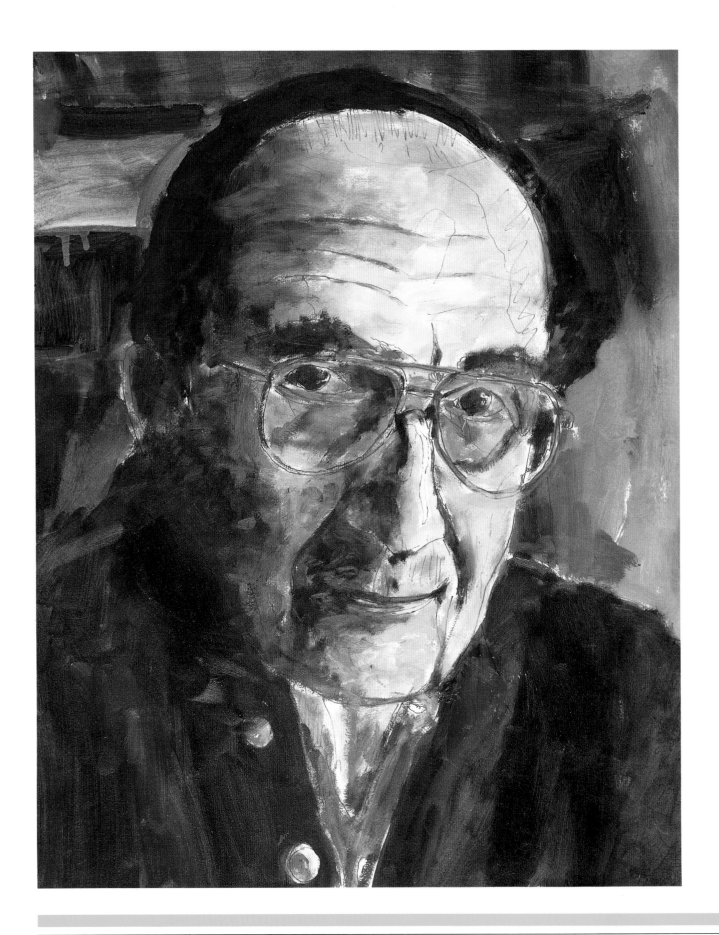

Dr. Salvador E. Luria, Nobel Laureate. 1984. Oil on paper, 19 x 15″. Collection Massachusetts Institute of Technology.

November 8 is designated Dunce Day to remember John Duns Scot, a medieval scholastic theologian who died on that day in 1308. Also known as "Dr. Subtilis," he and his followers, the Dunses, were both impervious to new knowledge and concerned with picayune technicalities.

It is a recurring theme in present educational circles, as it was in educational circles of the past, that we are confronted with an information explosion. This is certainly an exciting truth. As Lord Lister said, "You must always be students learning and unlearning till your life's end."

Although knowledge is a summation of facts, wisdom demands a critical assessment and simplification of these facts. A good teacher must assess what *not* to teach, a good student must learn what *not* to learn, and a good clinician must consider what tests *not* to order and what procedures *not* to perform. It must be appreciated that although information is provided by facts, tests, and studies, significant concepts can evolve and therapy can be prescribed without an impressive number of them. The patient with obstructive jaundice who has lost weight and has a palpable gallbladder and ultrasonographic demonstration of dilated intrahepatic and extrahepatic bile ducts does not need *both* a PTC and ERCP as well as a liver-spleen scan and gastrointestinal series. A diagnostic study that will not alter therapy is uncalled for and escalates medical costs.

William J. Mayo wrote, "One of the defects of our plan of education in this country is that we give too much attention to developing the memory and too little to developing the minds; we lay too much stress on acquiring knowledge and too little on the wise application of knowledge." We can all picture the dunce sitting in the corner wearing the characteristic conical cap. The desired antithesis could be drawn wearing an inverted cone that allows the mass of material that is poured into the wide mouth to be filtered so that only the appropriate is assimilated and invoked.

Flip the Foolscap

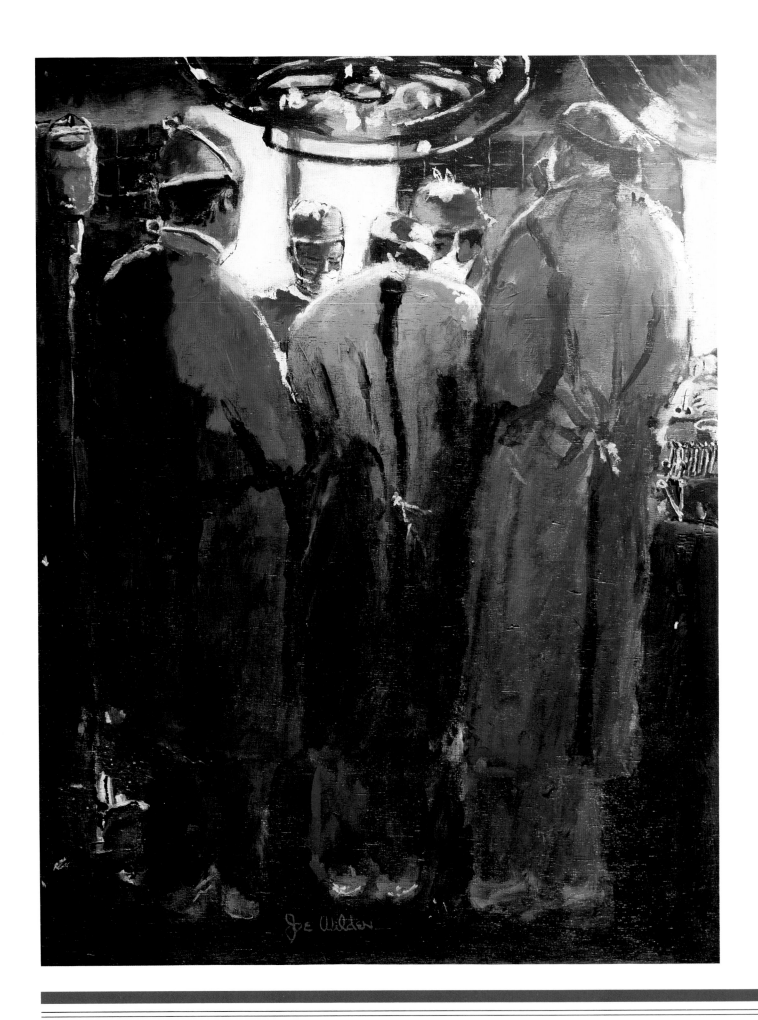

Five Surgeons and One Patient. 1989. Oil on panel, 24 x 18″.

*T*elevision instruction of colonoscopy is but a small example of the current educational tools that are destined to proliferate in the future. Video tape playbacks, perhaps even with slo-mo capabilities, will aid in the perfection of residents' surgical technique. Medical students will, to a greater extent, be exposed to the factual matter of medicine in quiet, detached library carrels using slides and tapes. Continuing medical education will be assimilated in stereo while commuting to and from work.

Even the most staid and conservative teachers would have to admit the favorable impact and potential of these electronic devices. However, a Lucifer does emerge from the luminescence of the diodes, and the circuitry has characteristics of the serpent of Eden.

The diabolic feature is that of disassociation from personalities—that is, pedagogues who provoke, teachers who titillate, and educators who excite. Theodor Billroth wrote, "A person may have learned a great deal and still be an exceedingly unskillful physician. The manner of dealing with patients . . . the student can learn only from immediate contact with the teacher whom he will unconsciously imitate."

That learning is catalyzed by interpersonal relations between students and teachers is obvious. An equally important stimulus is that which occurs between students themselves. Peter Mere Latham, the great teacher of medicine in early nineteenth century England, wrote, "I would wish to see the freest intercourse between pupils with a view to mutual instruction. You have it in your power to give infinite help to each other."

Machine-generated learning detaches and isolates the student at all levels. The soundproof carrel wall, the impersonal computer program, and the postgraduate lecture pondered in an automobile readily serve as shields that interrupt the combustive and excitative chain reaction vital to learning.

Thus, the application of modern and future teaching machines requires an extrinsic modulation to maintain the essence of strong personal stimuli. In truth, a single stimulating word from an inspiring teacher is worth a thousand pictures.

Personal Touch

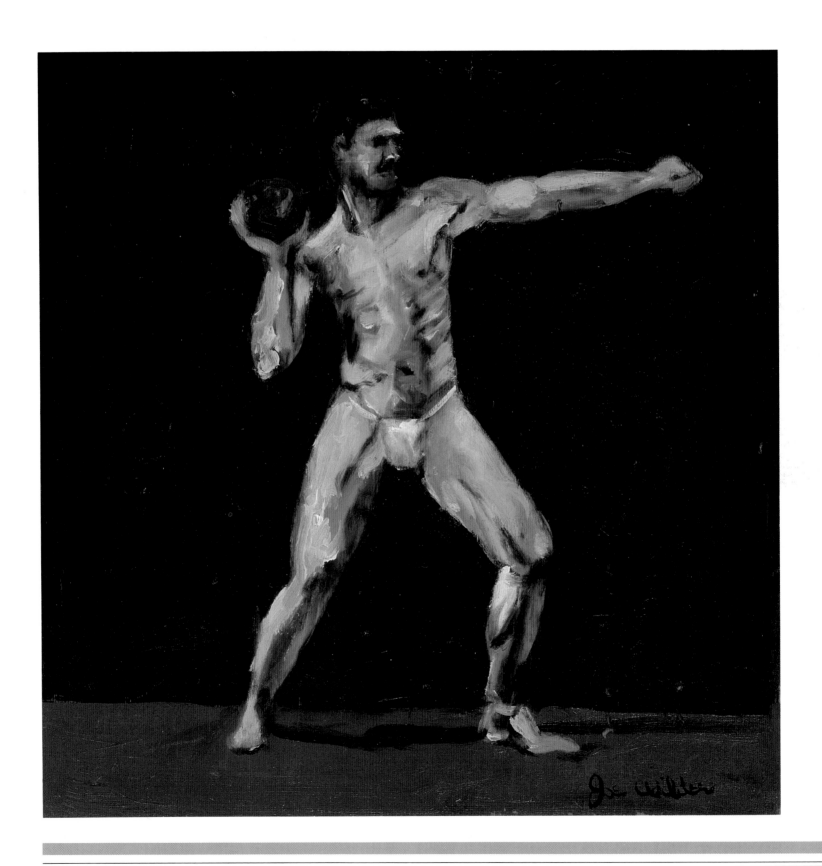

Shotputter, after Muybridge. 1986. Oil on panel, 12 x 12″.

A knowledge of anatomy has been, and will remain, the keystone of an operative procedure. The very word literally means "cut up," derived from the Greek *ana,* or up, and *tome,* or cut; the word could serve as an emblem for our profession. The current era of surgery has been dominated by extraordinary advances in surgical pathology and refinements in technology. Our understanding of surgical anatomy is inherited from past eras, and that heritage provides a skeleton for the dynamic progress in surgery brought about by a relatively recent understanding of surgical physiology.

The famous English explorer, John Smith, wrote in 1624, "As Geography without History seemeth as carkasse without motion, so History without Geography wandereth as vagrant without a certaine habitation." Along a similar but more pertinent line, Jean Fernel, the greatest French physician of the Renaissance, concluded that "Anatomy is to physiology as geography to history; it describes the theatre of events."

The modern curriculum provides a relatively abbreviated exposure to anatomy and a limited period for personal dissection of a cadaver. W. Somerset Maugham, the physician turned novelist, offered advice to first-year medical students in his book *Of Human Bondage:* "In anatomy it is better to have learned and lost than never to have learned at all." In reference to the swing away from the personal experience in dissecting, the great da Vinci's words should be heeded: "And you who think to reveal the figure of man in *words* . . . banish the idea from you, for the more minute the description the more you will confuse the mind."

In a medical era dominated by the excitement of molecular biology and the unraveling of basic biochemical events, anatomy has receded into a corner of concern. As a science, it is rarely regarded as exciting, and this is made manifest by the fact that most chairmen of departments of anatomy in modern medical schools have their prime interest in a field other than that which most of us would regard as classical anatomy.

It is true that the body of knowledge about anatomy has changed little since a 31-year-old by the name of Henry Gray published the first edition of his *Anatomy.* Continued expansion of surgery, however, has put an increasing demand on an appreciation of the development, structure, and anomalies of organs and segments of the body that are becoming the objects of operative extirpation or repair. Guy de Chauliac's fourteenth century aphorism, "A blind man works on wood the same way as a surgeon on the body when he is ignorant of anatomy," is even more meaningful today.

Sans Anatomy,
Blindness

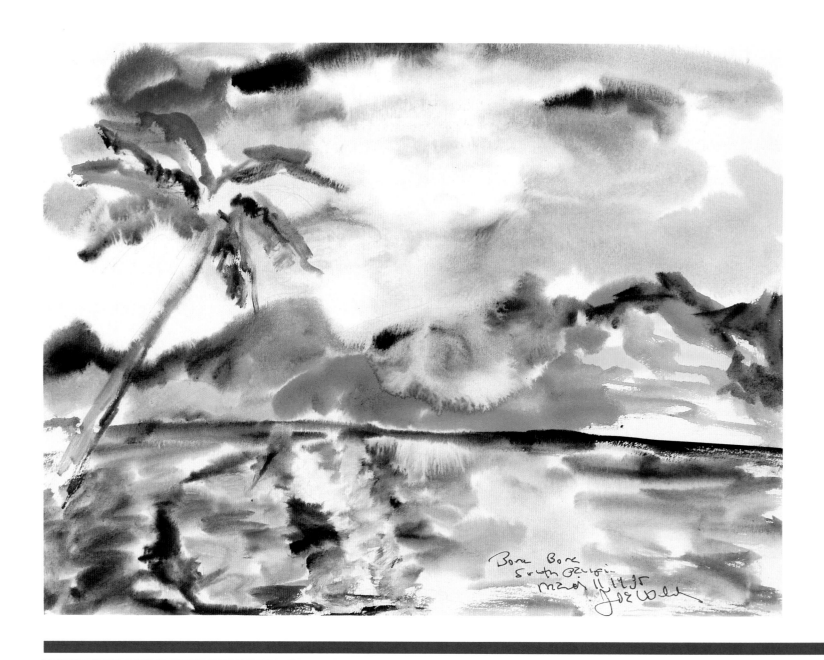

Bora Bora. 1985. Watercolor, 9 x 12″.

*T*he coming of age of consumerism has focused attention on the question of relicensure. How often has a physician or surgeon been asked by one of the laity, "How do you reconcile the fact that an airline pilot, who is responsible for the lives of passengers, requires periodic testing to maintain his or her license while members of the medical profession, which has as its specific commodity patients' lives and well-being, do not?"

The patient-consumer is asking for evidence that the physician to whom he entrusts his care has stayed current. This desiratum has long been a requisite of medical practice. The case has been stated by diverse men of greatness.

John Shaw Billings, distinguished surgeon in the Civil War, bibliographer, principal founder of the Surgeon General's Library, and planner and civil administrator of the New York Public Library, wrote in 1894, "The education of a doctor which goes on after his degree is, after all, the most important part of his education."

Sir William Osler, categorized by his former intern, Dean Wilbur T. Davison of Duke University, as physician, teacher, scientist, reformer, writer, and humanist, stated in an address delivered in 1900, "If the license to practice meant the completion of his education, how sad it would be for the practitioner, how distressing to his patients! More clearly than any other, the physician should illustrate the truth of Plato's saying that education is a lifelong process."

Karl Marx, a philosopher whose views I do not generally share, also voiced the concept when he said, "The education of most people ends upon graduation; that of the physician means a lifetime of incessant study."

I strongly support continuing education. Perhaps it is now appropriate for the Liaison Committee on Continuing Medical Education to be charged with the responsibility for assessing these courses and publishing an annual descriptive catalogue to aid physicians and surgeons in making appropriate choices. This suggestion is presented with full appreciation of the point emphasized by Dean George T. Harrell: "The physician's continuing education, whether he is a scientist practicing in a medical school or a general practitioner practicing in some rural area, is largely a process within himself, one he pursues on his own."

A Continuum

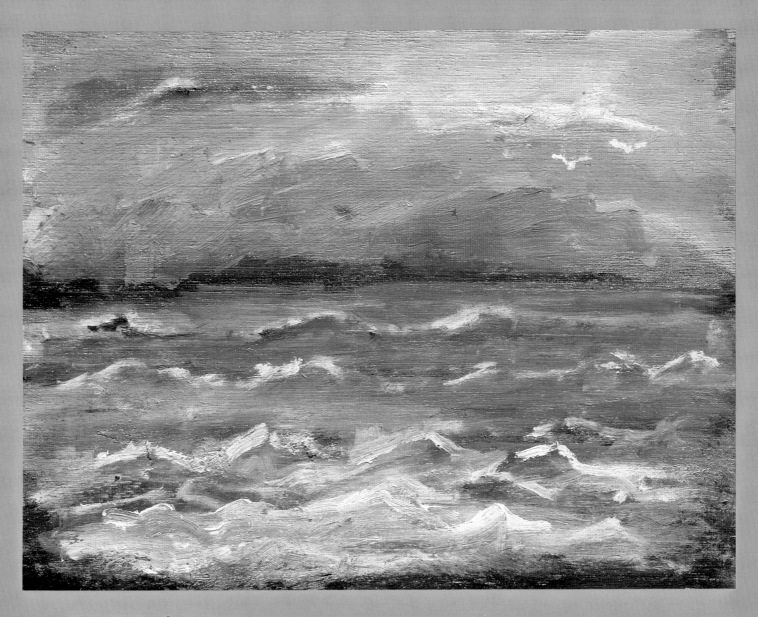

PART SIX

Obiter Dicta

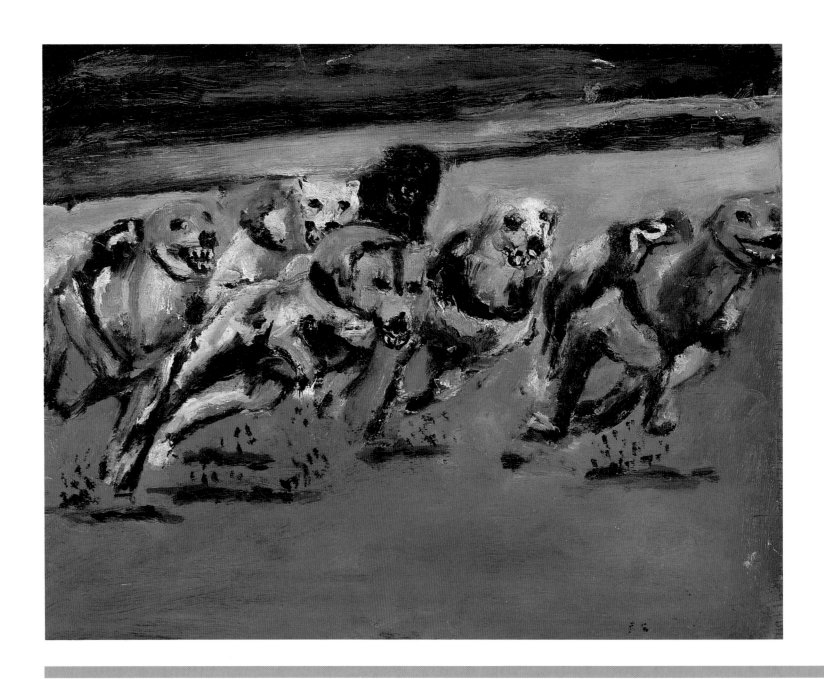

Dog Race. 1987. Oil on panel, 9 x 12″.

In 1811, J.F.D. Jones wrote, "The surgeon never suffers greater anxiety than when he is called upon to suppress a violent hemorrhage; and on no occasion is the reputation of his art so much at stake."

The Ebers papyrus gives evidence of the early recognition of the importance of hemostasis: "I will treat the disease with the knife, paying heed to the vessels." Celsus, in the first century A.D., proposed ligature of vessels, but as a matter of last resort. In the following century Galen recommended ligating arteries with Celtic linen, but his major impetus was his authoritative support of the Hippocratic dictum espousing the use of cautery. Before the sixteenth century, cauterization remained the dominant hemostatic device, with exceptions expressed by Ugo of Lucca and Henri de Mondeville, who wrote, "God did not exhaust all the creative power in making Galen."

But it was at the siege of Danvilliers in 1552 that the modern era of surgical hemostasis began when Ambroise Paré used the ligature in the course of an amputation and also used a bullet extractor, *bec de corbin,* to grasp the vessel, thus providing the ancestor of the modern hemostat. At another siege that took place at Besancon in 1674, Morel first introduced the tourniquet, which facilitated isolation of vessels for ligation.

The pathophysiology of hemostasis, the appreciation of coagulation, and the application of a scientific method to study the control of hemorrhage are all credited to practicing surgeons. In 1731, Jean-Louis Petit, who is better known for his screw tourniquet, was the first to conclude that hemorrhage is stopped by the formation of a coagulum or clot of blood (*caillot de sang*), which lies partly without and partly within the blood vessels. He also added that when hemorrhage is stopped by the application of a ligature, a clot is formed above the ligature. William Hewson, a surgeon who for a time was William Hunter's partner, localized the source of the fibrous network of clot to "coagulable lymph" in 1711, thus earning the accolade of the Father of Coagulation.

For the initiation of scientific methodology we must regard J.F.D. Jones's treatise on hemorrhage, published in Philadelphia in 1811; he described the experiments on arteries of the horse, dog, and ass, investigating "The Process Employed by Nature in Suppressing the Hemorrhage from Divided and Punctured Arteries, and on the Use of the Ligature; Concluding with Observations on Secondary Hemorrhage."

The simplicity of hemostasis, as stated in the *Aeneid*, "therewith the leach unwitting rinsed the wound and the pain fled, and all the blood was stayed" has been replaced by refinements of surgical hemostatic devices and manipulations of deficiencies in the coagulation process designed to make intraoperative bleeding a tolerable attendant and a less formidable opponent.

Besting the Beast

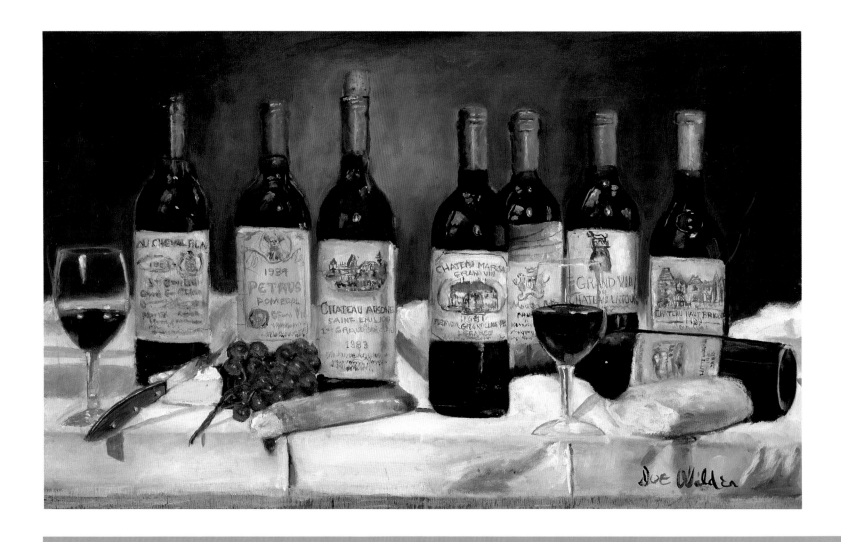

Bordeaux's First Growth. 1988. Oil on panel, 14 x 24″. Collection Morris W. Offit.

*C*redit for raising the curtain on the multiple acts directed toward the control or management of surgical infections must be granted to Joseph Lister. The man who is regarded as the greatest nineteenth century surgical scientist was the son of a wine merchant with an interest in microscopy who had developed an achromatic lens that allowed better definition of bacteria. Joseph Lister was appointed professor of surgery at the University of Glasgow when he was 33 years old but had to wait 2 years for hospital privileges because the hospital board regarded its institution as "curative and not educational." It was within the Glasgow Hospital that the famous trials with carbolic acid treatment of compound fractures were begun as a direct off-shoot of Louis Pasteur's studies on fermentation. Lister instilled carbolic acid into the wounds to provide antisepsis and sprayed the operative field, but he assiduously avoided scrubbing because he felt that it created crevices in which bacteria would thrive.

Credit for effecting control of surgical infections should also be given to the supporting players. F.C. Calvert, professor of chemistry in the Royal Institute of Manchester, was responsible for preparing carbolic acid in pure form, and he made it available at a moderate price. James Greenlees deserves recognition because it was the compound fracture of his leg that was dressed with putty impregnated carbolic acid in August 1865. The patient was discharged in 6 weeks with two functional legs, representing the first of Lister's successes following two previous failures with the same regimen.

Credit must also go to the editors of *Lancet* for printing six installments of a series of articles in 1867 entitled "On a New Method of Treating Compound Fractures, Abscess, Etc., With Observations on the Conditions of Suppuration." Eleven cases of compound fracture were reported in this review; only one patient required an amputation, and there was one death as a result of hemorrhage.

Initial contemporary audience reaction to Lister's therapeutic approach was not uniformly favorable. Lister's 2½-hour lecture evoked scepticism at the Philadelphia Medical Congress held in 1876 as part of the American Centennial. Credit should be given to James L. Cabell, professor of surgery and physiology at the University of Virginia, who presented a positive review of Lister's concepts in Volume I of the proceedings of the American Surgical Association. However, in the discussion of this article, J.W.S. Gouley of New York said, "I have always been a consistent anti-Listeric surgeon." E.M. Moore of Rochester, who was to become president of the American Surgical Association, felt that the carbolic spray contributed to death. And C.H. Mastin, another future president of the organization, indicated that surgeons in the state of Alabama had ceased to use Lister's method. Yet 8 years later, as president, he would extol Lister. As Lister himself stated, "Next to the promulgation of the truth, the best thing I can conceive that a man can do is the public recantation of an error."

Credits

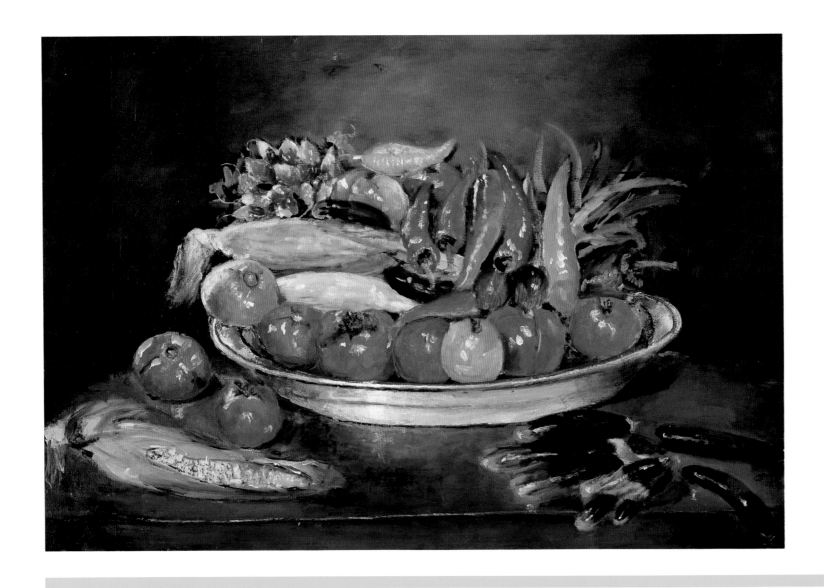

Celebration of November Vegetables. 1992. Oil on panel, 20 x 30″.

Nutrition is truly a twentieth century science, but the word was introduced in the sixteenth century and early contributions in the eighteenth century laid the groundwork for its evolution.

Lavoisier (1743-1794) usually is referred to as the Father of Nutrition because of his work on respiration, oxidation, and calorimetry. Two military surgeons also contributed significantly. The first clinical nutrition laboratory was established in 1753 on the HMS *Salisbury* by James Lind, who scientifically identified a cure for scurvy. In the early nineteenth century, William Beaumont studied the process of human digestion with his unique clinical investigations of Alexis St. Martin's gastric fistula. By the early nineteenth century, Magendie had revealed that the support of life of a dog required a source of nitrogen in the food.

Nutrition's older sister, Dietetics, has an even longer ancestry, dating to antiquity. The Greeks and Romans were concerned with the medical implications of diet. Lin Yutang stated, "The Chinese do not draw any distinction between food and medicine." Andrew Boorde, physician to Henry VIII in the early 16th century, wrote, "The chief physicke doth come from the kitchen." Lucretius, in the century before Christ, succinctly exclaimed: "Edo, ergo sum" (I eat, therefore I am).

Although we generally eat from habit and to satisfy metabolic needs, there are times that we eat for pleasure. Brillant-Savarin, who for a period of time in the late eighteenth century played violin in a New York theater orchestra, returned to Paris to become remembered for the epicurean dimension he added to the process by which we nourish ourselves. It was he who wrote in *Physiologie du Gout* (Physiology of Taste), "The discovery of a new dish is more beneficial to humanity than the discovery of a new star."

The substitution of palatal pleasure with nutrients that bypass the sensations of smell and taste is a modern event. Today, when parenteral nutrition has so significantly modified our care of patients, we can evoke the thirteenth century observation of Roger Bacon: "If the elements should be prepared and purified in some mixture so that there would be action of one element on another but so that they would be reduced to pure simplicity . . . the status quo of body could be maintained."

Food for Thought

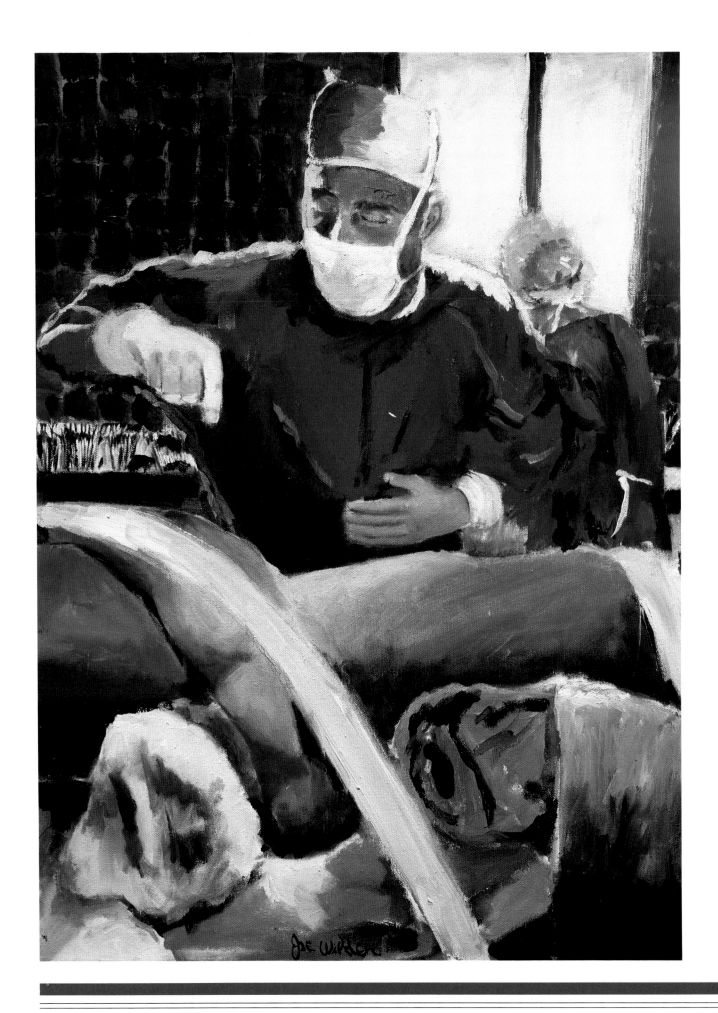

Positioning Patient. 1987. Oil on canvas, 24 x 18″.

I am not a trauma surgeon or a member of the American Association for the Surgery of Trauma, but I regard trauma as an optimal focus in the education of students of surgery. Compressed into a relatively short time for each clinical situation, a diagnosis must be entertained and acted on rapidly and the effects of treatment evaluated. A diversity of systems, organs, lesions, and problems may be addressed. The field of trauma is a uniquely surgical arena unfettered by territorial battles with other disciplines—an educational haven if not a heaven.

An often quoted Oslerian statement is "Know syphilis in all its manifestations and relations and all things clinical will be known unto you." An analogy could be "Know trauma in all its manifestations and complications and all surgical principles will be known unto you." The chronicles of surgical history show that many advances were made as a consequence of managing war wounds. Hippocrates wrote, "He who wishes to be a surgeon should go to war." The oldest record of surgical teaching, the Smith Papyrus, focuses on the management of wounds. The first major contribution of Theodor Billroth was his 1859 treatise on the management of gunshot wounds. The biographer of Alexis Carrel suggests that the pioneering work in vascular anastomosis was stimulated by the death of French President Sadi Carnot, who exsanguinated from a lacerated portal vein.

The management of trauma, be it blood vessels, bones, brain, or viscera, is the soil of surgery from which the principles have grown for treatment of inflammatory, degenerative, and malignant processes. In the past I have quoted James Henry Breasted, the translator of the Papyrus: "The Edwin Smith Papyrus has revealed to us an ancient Egyptian *surgeon* [in his management of traumatized patients] in contrast with the physician, as a man with the ability to observe, to draw conclusions from his observations, and thus, within the limitations of his age, to maintain a scientific attitude of mind."

The Teaching Tool

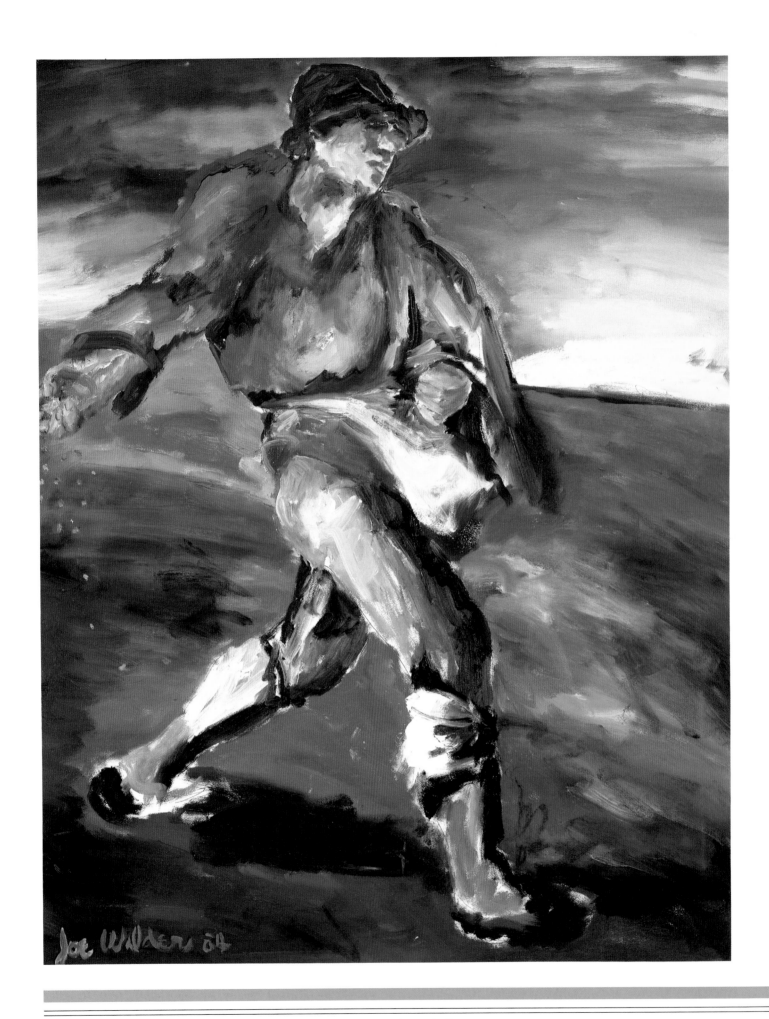

Millet's Sower. 1984. Oil on canvas, 30 x 24″. Collection Dr. Andrew Karlin.

The Biblical statement of Job, "My skin is black upon me and my bones are burnt with heat," indicates the magnitude of the local problems associated with burns. No other insult can so profoundly destroy anatomic structures and alter physiologic functions. The extent the pendulum swings regarding the management of burn wounds has passed through the 180-degree arc several times.

In the late eighteenth and early nineteenth century, two major polarized camps championed either cold therapy or the application of heat. Those extolling the virtues of cold, such as Mr H. Earle, surgeon to St. Bartholomew's Hospital, whose lectures appeared in the *London Medical Gazette* of 1830, point out that this approach was advocated by Rhazes and Avicenna. On the other hand, the most famous eighteenth century essay on burns, written in 1797 by Edward Kentish, advocated applying the same stimulus as that which caused the burn—that is, heat. This approach could have invoked the support of Aristotle and Shakespeare: "Fire cools fire within the scorched veins of one new burnt."

It is both reassuring and disturbing to realize that whenever great minds are polarized on a definitive therapeutic approach, half are always wrong.

John Hunter's eighteenth century *Lecture on the Principles of Surgery* gives evidence of the wisdom of the man. "Many wounds ought to be allowed to scab in which this process is now prevented; and this arises, I believe, from the conceit of surgeons who think themselves possessed of powers superior to nature and therefore have introduced the practice of making sores of all wounds. The mode of assisting the cure of wounds by permitting a scab to form is likewise applicable, in some cases, to that species of accident where the parts have not only been lacerated but deprived of life. . . . This practice is the very best for burns and scalds."

When therapeutic zealots are culled and vested interest discounted, the pendulum most frequently finds a midline position as expressed by Jacob Bigelow in Volume I of the *New England Journal of Medicine and Surgery* of 1812, "After considering at length the opposite extremes of treatment which have been adopted; results of both reason and experiments appears to be, that the two extremes are like injudicious, when pursued in their full extent; and neither of them suited to the varieties of burns and of constitutions. An intermediate plan of treatment, which shall vary according to circumstances, and be dependent on the degree and state of disease, is undoubtedly the most deserving of attention."

Perhaps the most meaningful statement in Kentish's *Essay on Burns* is one to which all clinical investigators should pay reverence before extolling the virtues of a given therapeutic approach: "It falls to the lot of few men to appreciate properly the effects of various modes of treatment in a particular disease; for if the patient recovers whatever was the treatment whether good or bad we flatter ourselves it was the effect of our superior merit in conducting the disease; but future experiments may convince us that the recovery of which we so vainly boasted was a victory of nature over the malpractice of art."

The Pendulum Rests

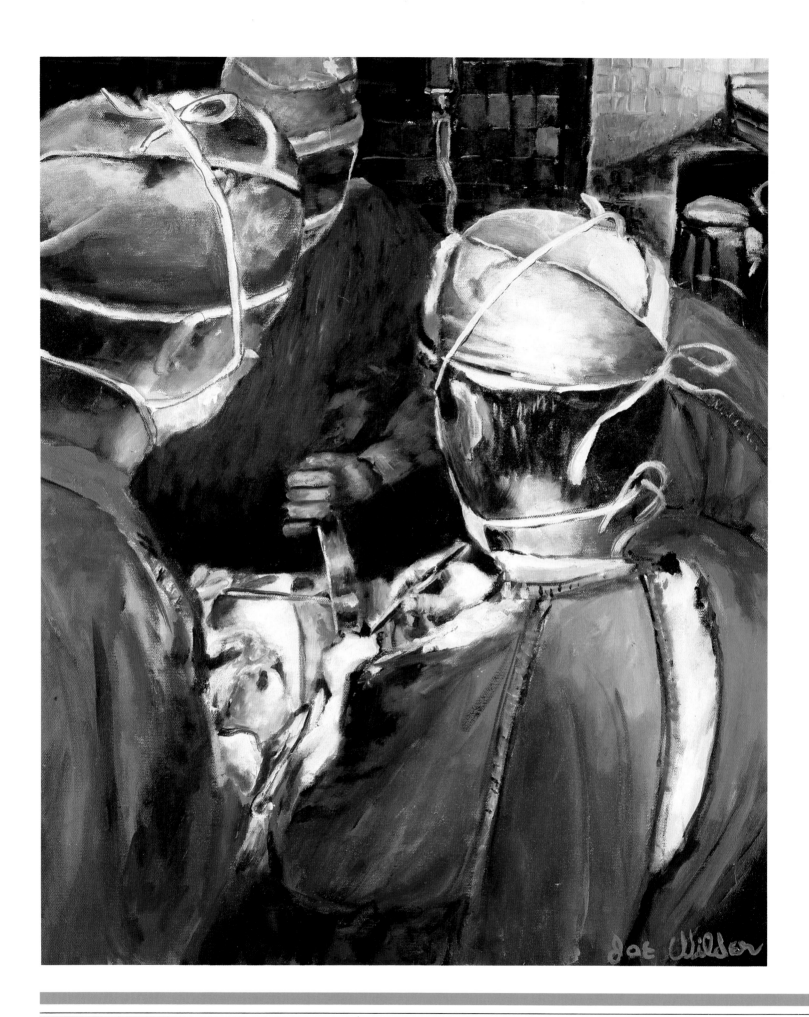

Sharp Dissection. 1987. Oil on canvas, 24 x 20″. Collection of Nick Wilder.

As recently as 25 years ago, there was a story told of a patient who died subsequent to an extensive resection by a cancer surgeon; the autopsy report stated that there was insufficient material for pathologic evaluation. Until recently, the essence of surgical management of patients with malignant tumors was a zealous excision of large amounts of tissue beyond the visible border of the lesion. Halsted is reported to have said, "The surgeon who removes a breast with a malignant tumor should be the mortal enemy of the one who will be closing the wound," indicating that the extent of resection should in no way be compromised.

The surgeon of today appreciates that the function of a "cancer operation" is to remove a lesion that one hopes is contained. Extending the resection to greater distances beyond the tumor adds little. Statistical analysis has shown that total gastrectomy does not improve the survival of patients with antral carcinoma compared with patients who have had partial gastrectomy; total pancreatectomy is no better than partial pancreatectomy for ductal carcinoma. The radical mastectomy and extended radical mastectomy techniques that were employed in the 1950s, 1960s, and early 1970s are now regarded as the dinosaurs in the evolution of operations for breast cancer.

In *Doctors Versus Folks,* Robert Tuttle Morris wrote, "The greatest triumph for surgery today . . . lies in finding ways for avoiding surgery," and "Allow patients to escape with the slightest attack of surgery your skill can supply." In an atmosphere of holistic care that the surgeon should provide, Logan Clendening's statement, "Surgery does the ideal thing—it separates the patient from the disease. It puts the patient back to bed and the disease in the bottle," requires modification. Although the goal of putting all the disease in a bottle remains, the other goal is to return the patient to near normalcy rather than to a bedridden or compromised lifestyle. A patient, not a tumor, is the focus of an operation.

Corporal Conservation

137

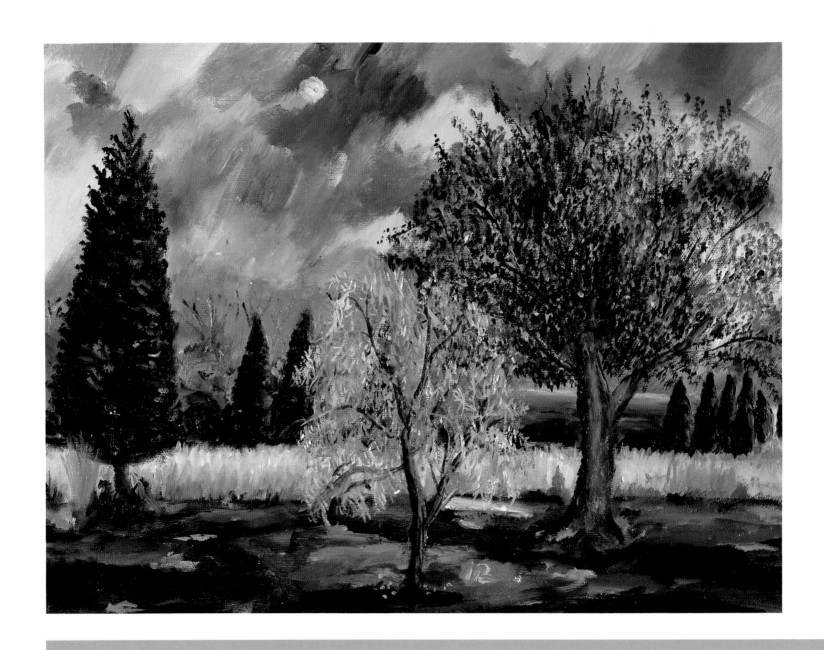

Juniper Tree, Apple Tree, Willow Tree. 1980. Oil on canvas, 12 x 16″.

*H*ernia, a disorder that was neglected by Hippocrates in his writings, derives from the Greek term *hernios,* meaning a branch or offshoot of a tree. The very term stresses the swelling and neglects the fascial defect. Chaucer also focused on the element of protrusion as evidenced by his phrase, "horrible swollen members that semeth like the maladie of Hirnia." The remarkable perception of the pathology was demonstrated by Andrew Boorde in the mid-sixteenth century when he wrote, "There be thre kindes named . . . a wateryshe herny, a wyndy hernye, a fleshely herny."

The history related to the surgical management of inguinal hernias is most intriguing. Celsus in the first century A.D. emphasized the ligation of the base of the protrusion and essentially disregarded repair of the canal. In the Middle Ages attention continued to be focused on the sac (the famous Frère Jacques is said to have operated on more than 2000 hernias); it was not until the pre-Listerian contributions of Scarpa, Cooper, and Hesselbach that the importance of the floor of the inguinal canal was appreciated. Edoardo Bassini generally is credited as being the first person to combine ligation of the sac with a physiologic reconstruction of the inguinal canal. However, American surgeons can well be proud to recognize Dr. Henry O. Marcy of Boston. This man, generally overlooked as a surgical great, was the first American pupil of Lister and the first to use absorbable sutures, specifically the kangaroo tendon, for repair of an inguinal hernia. Actually, he preempted Bassini in describing an operation that sequentially transfixed the neck of the cord, removed the redundant part, and used the transversalis fascia to reconstruct the posterior wall.

Today hernia repair occupies the position of a benchmark procedure with which all other surgical efforts are compared. This would be regarded as more than appropriate by Sir Astley Cooper, who introduced his famous folio publication on hernia, published in 1804, with the statement, "No disease of the human body, belonging to the province of the surgeon, requires in its treatment a greater combination of accurate anatomical knowledge, with surgical skill, than hernia in all its variety."

Benchmark Bulge

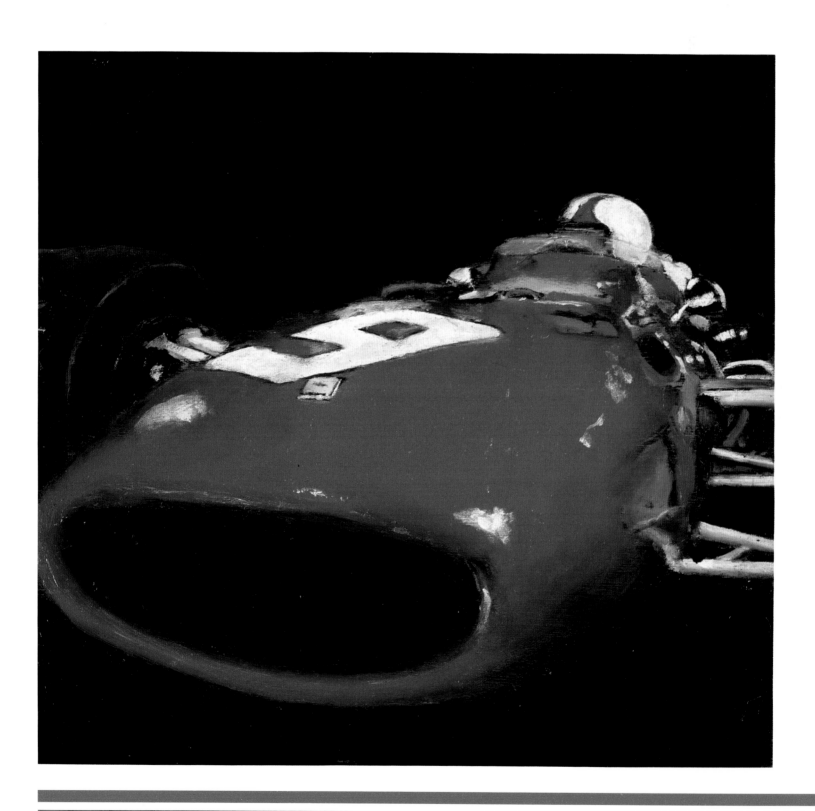

Ferrari No. 9. 1985. Oil on panel, 13 x 14". Collection William Burden.

The word "thyroid" is derived from Greek, meaning shield, but it was actually first used to refer to the cartilage bearing that name. The name was applied to the gland itself by Thomas Wharton, who in 1659 called it "thyreodea." Goiter was a subject of interest in antiquity; early Egyptian carvings provide evidence of its existence. In 1600 B.C., the Chinese appreciated the ameliorative effects of burnt sponge and seaweed on goiter. In the thirteenth century, Marco Polo said of the Chinese in certain regions where he traveled, "They are in general affected with tumors on the throat occasioned by the nature of the water which they drink." In the tenth century *Book of Haly Abbas* it says, "For goiter in which such medication is of no avail, surgery is necessary." The first successful thyroidectomy on record appears to have been performed about 952 A.D. by Albucasin, a Moor physician. Guy de Chauliac, in the fourteenth century, advised removal of the diseased gland.

Professor Emil Theodor Kocher of Berne, Switzerland, devoted major efforts to the study of the thyroid gland. He observed that removal of the thyroid produced myxedema; his research placed thyroid surgery on a sound basis. Consequently, in 1909 he became the first surgeon to receive the Nobel Prize. Kocher reported more than 2000 thyroidectomies performed in the nineteenth century, with a 4.5% mortality. He continually emphasized that some functioning gland be left and that ligature of the arteries of the remaining gland should be avoided.

Halsted wrote that "the extirpation of the thyroid gland for goiter typifies, perhaps better than any operation, the supreme triumph of the surgeon's art." Many of the most distinguished clinics in our country (Mayo, Lahey, Cleveland) evolved and flourished to a large extent based on experiences with thyroidectomy.

But the gland that is so important to the surgeon has not gained the respect of all. H.L. Mencken, in a 1922 letter to Theodore Dreiser, wrote, "When I die my kidneys go to the municipal museum of Altoona, Pa., and my liver to Oberlin College, but it would take much eloquence to make me leave even my thyroid gland to Milwaukee."

Emblems on a Shield

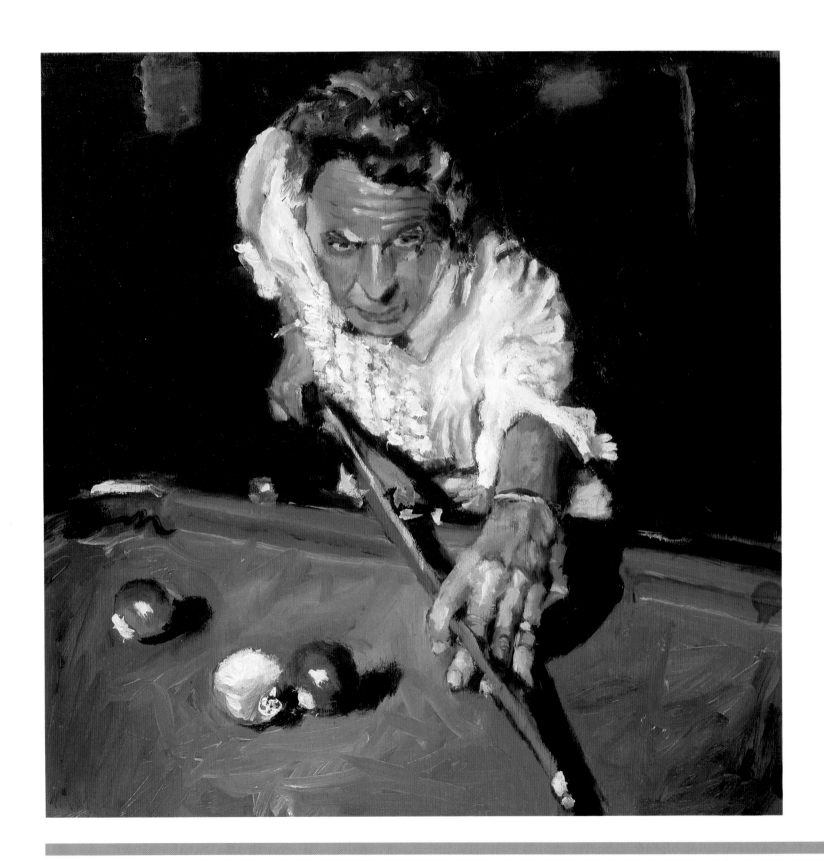

Pool Champion Milton Robertson. 1985. Oil on panel, 12 x 12″. Collection Morris W. Offit.

The application of endoscopy to the gastrointestinal tract, be it peroral or peranal, has elevated the diagnosis of alimentary tract diseases to a level of precision and refinement previously restricted to the urinary tract. No longer must deductive reasoning or guesswork be used to find the cause of bleeding in cirrhotic patients; in most cases this can be determined by esophagoscopy and gastroscopy. Endoscopic retrograde cholangiopancreatography (ERCP) has refined the diagnosis of disorders of the biliary tract and pancreas. Sigmoidoscopy and its extension of colonoscopy have major diagnostic and therapeutic consequences.

Forty-six years ago, the dramatic text of George S. Chappell and surrealistic drawings of cartoonist O. Soglow in *Through the Alimentary Canal With Gun and Camera* (New York, Dover Publications) foreshadowed the present in Jules Verne fashion. This book is recommended as a delightful and remarkable expedition. Persisting in the humorist's pathway, we might suggest that esophagoscopy, gastroscopy, and ERCP, with the wonders of pathology they uncover, be regarded as "per-awe-all" rather than peroral studies. To complete the punster's lexicon, sigmoidoscopy and colonoscopy, with their potential yield, might be called "perennial" rather than peranal.

Quo vadis? To what greater heights will the inventive mind carry our visual investigations? Now available in prototype and being optically refined is an adaptation of the simple hypodermic needle, which has been converted successfully to an endoscope to permit reasonable visualization of previously hidden areas. By this means, for example, the interior of a renal cyst can be punctured and the cyst wall assessed. Improved light sources and flushing systems may very well permit luminal evaluation of blood vessels and direct definition of intra-arterial and intravenous lesions.

Diagnostic endoscopy doubtless will become a jousting ground for internists and surgeons, since it provides intellectual satisfaction, important information, and economic compensation. For the physicians who participate—and it is true that significant contributions to the art and science of endoscopy have been made by physicians— the designation "internist" finally may become justified.

Visual Investigations

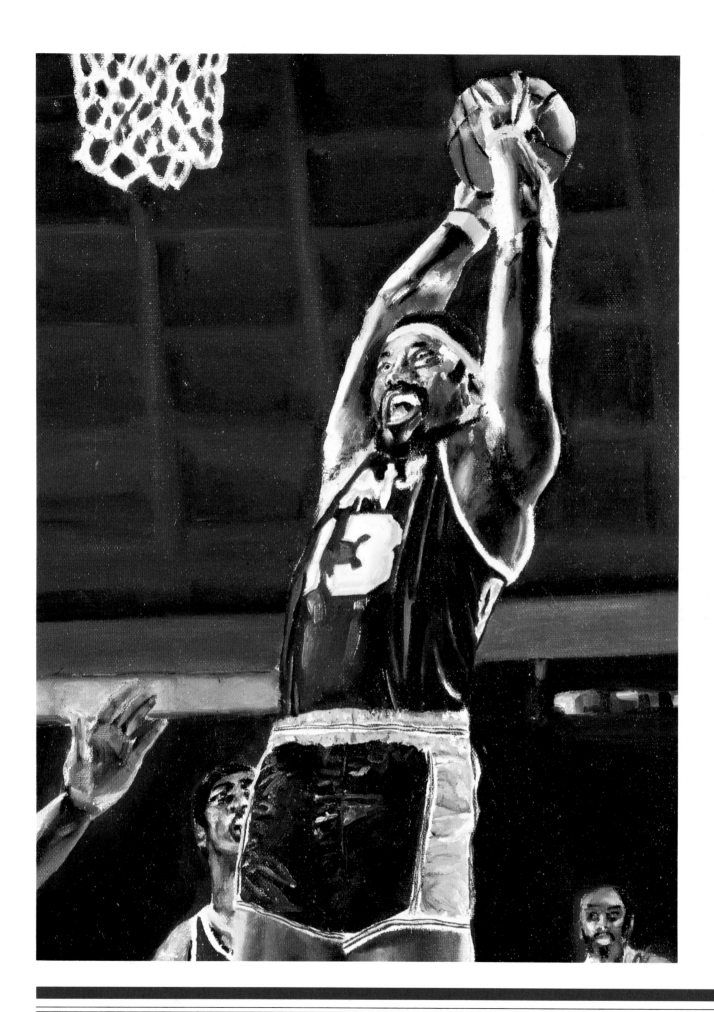

Wilt Chamberlain. 1975. Oil on canvas, 16 x 12″. Collection Dr. Richard Gibbs.

Saint Fiacre, the patron saint of those afflicted with hemorrhoids, would have been pleased to learn that the first surgical specialty hospital was dedicated to the management of anal disorders. The major modern contribution associated with that hospital is in preserving fecal continency. The saga began more than 150 years ago.

The nineteenth century in England was characterized by the progress of "the specialist" movement. Before that time the only two conditions that received special treatment in specialty hospitals were lunacy and leprosy. In 1805, the London Dispensary was founded for the relief of the poor afflicted with eye disease. In 1814, the Royal Hospital for Disease of the Chest was established for the treatment of consumption. In 1835, St. Mark's Hospital became the first surgical specialty hospital. Dr. Frederick Salmon founded the institution that bore the title "St. Mark's Hospital for Fistula." That fistula-in-ano should have constituted the focus for the establishment for the first surgical hospital is distinctly appropriate. In the fourteenth century, John of Arderne required at least 100 shillings for a successful operation for anal fistula, 40 British pounds for the well-to-do, and 40 pounds and life annuity of 100 shillings for the wealthy. At that time, the ordinary laborer earned one penny a day.

In 1686, Louis XIV, the Sun King, had fistula-in-ano successfully operated on by Charles-Francois Felix. The success of this procedure had a lasting effect on the status of surgery. Shortly after the operation, a series of royal decrees extended the privileges of barber-surgeons so that they were able to operate on dead bodies and treat wounds. In 1694, the amphitheater of St. Come was constructed and eventually became the home of the French Academy of Surgery in 1731.

In *All's Well That Ends Well*, Shakespeare wrote, "What is it, my good lord, the King languishes of?" "A fistula, my lord." All has truly ended well—from fistula to recognition of surgery, to establishment of a hospital concerned with anal disorders to extension of interest of that hospital to diseases of the colon and rectum, and to development in that hospital of a procedure that preserves anal function and obviates the creation of a stoma.

Painful to Propitious

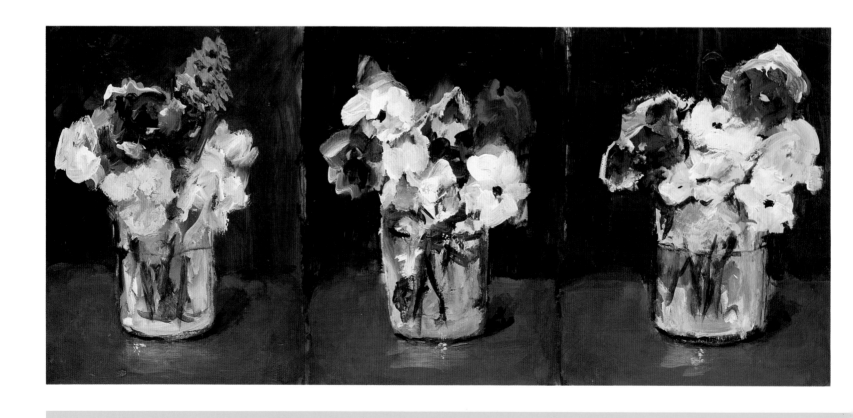

Pansies Triptych. 1992. Oil on wood, 8 x 20″. Collection Cynthia Wilder.

In the Book of Judges, Eglon, the King of Moab, was stabbed "and his dirt ran out and he died," suggesting that all such intestinal wounds are fatal. In extreme cases if "iliac passion," a term applied to intestinal obstruction, Praxagoras of Cos made an incision over the swelling of a strangulated hernia and cut into the bowel to establish an artificial anus.

Significant contributions concerning stomas were made in the eighteenth century. The first recorded suggestion for enterostomy is that of Littre, reported in 1710. Littre suggested the performance of an enterostomy in a patient with imperforate anus. The idea did not achieve fruition until 1776, when Pillore, a surgeon at Rouen, performed a cecostomy for cancer. Dubois applied Littre's specific suggestion in 1783, performing a colostomy in a child with an imperforate anus.

The real origin of colostomy is credited to Duret, who performed the operation in 1793 for a case of imperforate anus in a child 3 days old; the patient lived to the age of 45. In Duret's account, several extraordinary statements appear. The surgeon pointed out that "to give me confidence in this most extraordinary procedure, I performed it upon a dead body of a child of 15 days." He attempted a lumbar approach, hoping that he could remain extraperitoneal, but rapidly recognized that the lateral areas of the colon are peritonealized in a child. It was for this reason that the iliac approach was adopted. He wrote that Celsus' axiom, "It is better to employ a doubtful remedy than to condemn the patient in certain death," applied in this case. Duret secured the bowel by a suture in the mesocolon to obviate retraction, described prolapse on the sixth postoperative day, and used the artificial anus as a stoma through which an enema was performed to effect passage of stool.

In 1797, Professor Fine, in Geneva, performed a transverse colostomy in a 63-year-old woman for an obstruction caused by cancer of the rectum. He actually had intended to open the ileum, and it was only at autopsy 3 months later that he discovered he had performed a transverse colostomy. Colostomy was advanced to a proper place in surgery by Amussat of Paris, who collected the statistics of all cases from 1776 to his own first case in 1839. Over the 63 years there were 29 cases; 20 of these patients died. In a series of resections, he demonstrated that the peritoneal reflections of the colon in the lumbar region would permit an extraperitoneal lumbar approach. He concluded with the statement, "An artificial anus, it is true, is a grave infirmity, but is not insupportable."

Certainly the modern innovations in stoma surgery represent refinements, but it is essential, and humbling, to focus on the courageous steps taken by our surgical progenitors. This supports the aphorism, "All knowledge is but a remembrance and all discovery but a forgetting."

Archeology of an Aperture

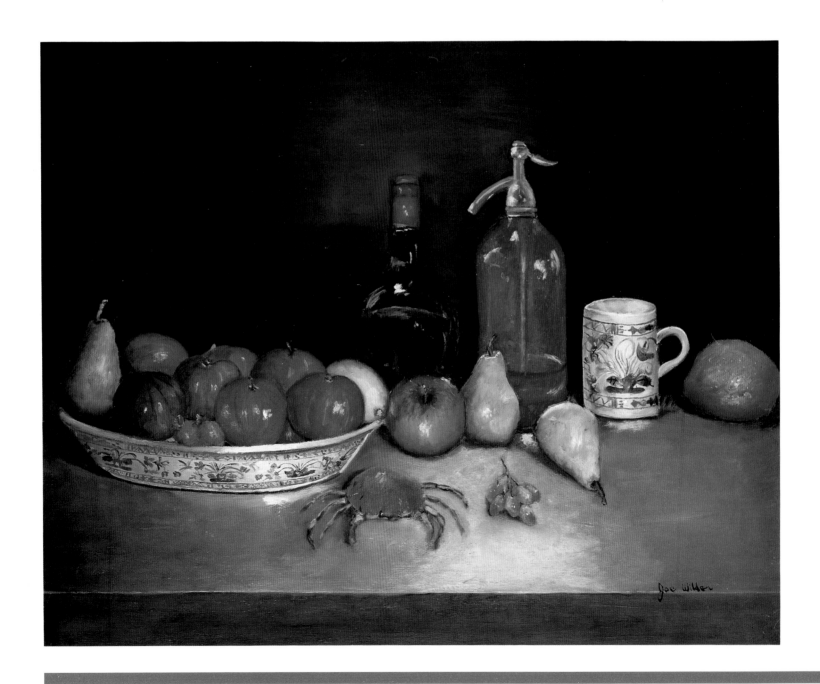

Still Life With Crab. 1983. Oil on canvas, 24 x 30".

The "organ of mystery" was the designation assigned to the spleen by Galen. In pre-Galenic times, Plato wrote, "The neighboring organ (the spleen) is situated on the left-hand side and is constructed with a view of keeping the liver bright and pure—like a napkin, always ready, prepared, and a hand to clean the mirror."

The spleen was one of Shakespeare's favorite organs and appears throughout his writings. Although it had previously been regarded as an organ of melancholy, the Bard used it in diverse ways exemplifying amusement, delight, merriment, whim or caprice, irritability, peevishness, impetuosity, and ill temper—in other words, an organ for all seasons. In *Twelfth Night* appears, "If you desire a spleene and will laugh yourself into stitches, follow me." In *Julius Caesar* the organ takes on a different profile: "You shal digest the venom of your spleene, though it do split you." What is undoubtedly the earliest reference to accessory spleens appears in *Venus and Adonis:* "A thousand spleens bear her a thousand days."

The first report chronicling successful treatment of splenic trauma is credited to Franciscus Rosetti, who in 1599 described a Dr. Viard's removal of a spleen that was protruding through the wound. In 1735, John Ferguson of Ireland performed a partial splenectomy on a protruded spleen and returned the remainder of the organ to the peritoneal cavity. The first splenectomy for trauma in the United States was carried out by a Royal Navy surgeon, who removed the spleen from a Mexican in California.

Splenic preservation is generally considered to be a modern concept, but salvage of a traumatized spleen was first reported by Parlavecchio in 1893. In 1895, the Russian surgeon, Zikoff, was the first to successfully suture a lacerated spleen. The change in attitude regarding the management of splenic trauma is in accord with Voltaire's definition of the physician's role: "To preserve and renew is almost as noble as to create." In the realm of nonoperative management, in 1881 Billroth reported the autopsy findings of a patient who died from a head injury and indicated that there was a splenic injury that "might have healed completely."

The contributions to the management of splenic trauma from around the globe reaffirm the international comradery of medicine. As Sir William Osler stated in his address on Chauvinism in Medicine: "What I inveigh against is a cursed spirit of intolerance, conceived in distrust and bred in ignorance, that makes the mental attitude perennially antagonistic, even bitterly antagonistic to everything foreign, that subordinates everywhere the race to the nation, forgetting the higher claims of human brotherhood."

Organ of Mystery

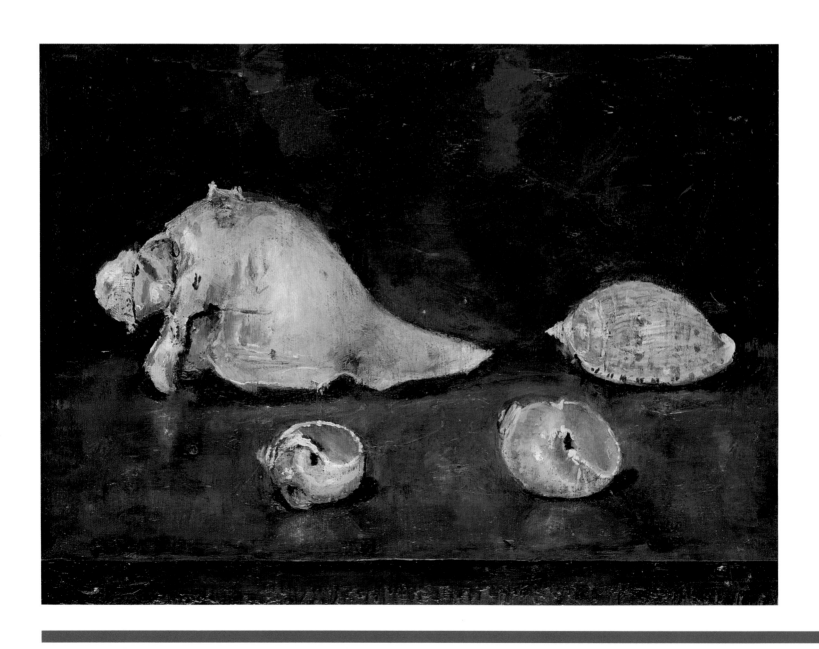

Four Ancient Seashells. 1990. Oil on panel, 11 x 15″.

The biliary calculus is the surgeon's gemstone. These small pebbles generate 750,000 cholecystectomies in North America each year. Thus historical review related to these concretions should strike a meaningful tone.

Nearly 30 calculi were found in the gallbladder of the mummy of a priestess of Amenen in the twenty-first Egyptian dynasty (c. 1500 B.C.), yet the ancient Greeks were curiously silent about gallstones. It was Trallianus in the sixth century who first made definite reference to gallstones, and by the sixteenth century both Vesalius and Fallopius described biliary calculi present in dissected bodies. At about the same time, the codification of the Talmud, with reference to dietary laws, incorporated a distinction between two types of calculi: "If hard things are found in the gallbladder, which are like the pits of dates, without sharp edges, the animal is kosher; but if the edges are sharp as in the pits of olives, the animal is *terefah* (unfit for eating)."

In the sixteenth century Jean Fernel, physician to the King of France, emphasized for the first time the importance of the role of stasis in the formation of biliary calculi; it was he who provided the first account of the clinical symptoms produced by these stones. Paracelsus, father of the metabolic theory of stone formation, proclaimed in his 1616 Doctrine of Tartarus that impure material ingested for nourishment might precipitate in the biliary passages. By 1740 Pouilletier de la Salle's work isolating cholesterol established a basis for the description of Vicq d'Azyr of two types of gallstones—those composed of cholesterol and those which additionally contained bile pigment. The last etiologic factor contributing to the formation of calculi was proposed by Morgagni; in 1767 he described glands in the gallbladder wall and indicated as the cause of gallstones the consequent inflammation of these glands.

Jean Louis Petit, regarded as the Father of Gallbladder Surgery, suggested in 1733 that the diagnosis of a large, inflamed gallbladder adherent to the anterior wall necessitated evacuation of the pus and removal of the stones. To the consternation of his peers, Petit successfully carried out this procedure in 1743.

It was not a physician but rather a German chemist, J.L.W. Tudichum, who first suggested a surgical approach for calculous disease. He proposed a two-stage procedure, suturing the gallbladder to the abdominal wall in the first stage and in the second stage, after the gallbladder was adherent to the parietal peritoneum, performing a cholecystotomy and removing the stones.

The first elective operation on the gallbladder took place June 15, 1867, on the third floor of a drug company in downtown Indianapolis. John Stough Bobbs, the first

Calculations

professor of surgery of the Indiana Medical College, operated on a 32-year-old woman with a large abdominal mass. Under chloroform anesthesia, he entered the gallbladder and removed many calculi and serous fluid. He palpated a retained stone in the region of the cystic duct. He then closed the cholecystotomy, an action that today would be firmly criticized. The patient, however, lived 45 years without complaints about her biliary tract and died of arteriosclerosis. The first planned cholecystostomy was performed by James Marion Sims in 1878, but unfortunately, the patient died on the eighth postoperative day.

A statement in the 1882 article by Carl Langenbuch, describing the first successful planned cholecystectomy, is particularly pertinent in the current practice of alternative dissolution therapy and lithotripsy: "The gallbladder should be removed not because it contains stones, but because it forms them."

A review of the history of illness in notable figures supports the role of surgical intervention. Alexander the Great is thought to have succumbed at age 34 to the consequences of acute cholecystitis and subsequent peritonitis. Sir Walter Scott agonized repeatedly from biliary colic, and General Douglas MacArthur elected to neglect common duct stones so long that secondary biliary cirrhosis and consequent portal hypertension ensued.

The word "calculus" is the diminutive of the Latin word *calx,* meaning stone. Calculus is also used to define a mathematical science—so named because of the little stones used in mathematical exercises performed on an ancient abacus. Management of biliary calculi should be based on an assessment of "calculated" risks.

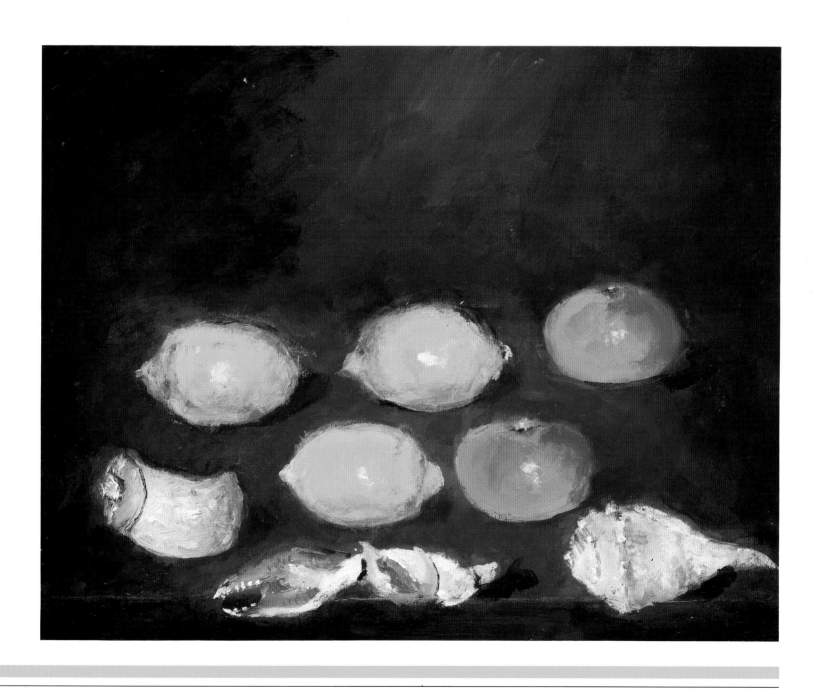

153   *Seashells, Fruit, and Crab Claw.* 1992. Oil on wood, 12 x 16″.

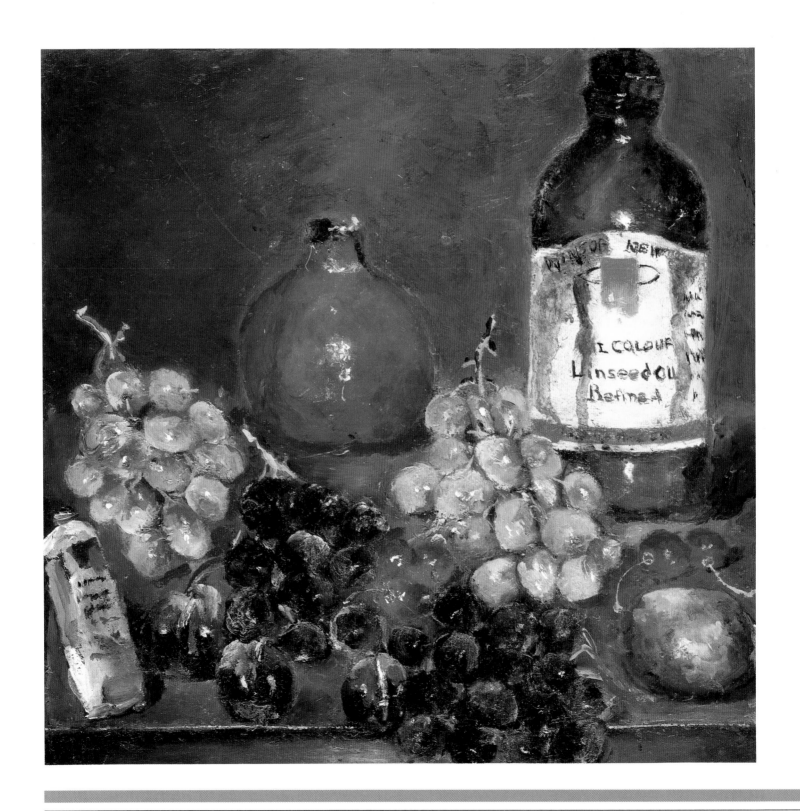

Grapes, Linseed Oil, Cherries, Lime, Pomegranate, and Oil Paint. 1990. Oil on panel, 12 x 12″.

During my internship, ligation of varicose veins was the procedure on which I whetted my scalpel, and the application of the Unna paste boot my domain. Many of the attitudes about aggressive surgery have been mollified since then, and operative procedures often have been replaced by sclerotherapy. But varicose veins remains one of the most common ailments of Western people, and as such merits historical consideration.

The Ebers Papyrus (c. 1550 B.C.) advised against an operation for varicose veins. Hippocrates ascribed leg ulcers to varicose veins, prescribed avoidance of standing, and also described compressive bandages. Plutarch, in his *Lives,* chronicles the case of Caius Marius, a Roman tyrant in the first century B.C. Following an operation on varicose veins in one of his legs, he declined the procedure on the other side because of intense pain.

Pertaining to the management of ulcer specifically, Celsus prescribed the use of plaster of paris and linen roller bandages. In the seventeenth and eighteenth centuries and in the early nineteenth century, when varices were thought to be caused by melancholic blood, it was widely held that ulcers were salutary and were best not treated. Richard Wiseman, Sergeant-Chirurgian to Charles II, was the first physician to relate leg ulcers to varicose veins. In 1676, he introduced the term "varicose ulcer" and devised a compressive leather stocking. Between the times of Celsus and Wiseman, others had advised compression as treatment for varicose ulcers. Henri de Mondeville, in the early fourteenth century, thought pressure was advantageous, since it would drive back the "evil humors." Guy de Chauliac later in that century, employed plaster of paris. The great Ambroise Paré in 1553 cured the ulcer of his captor: "Roule the leg, beginning at the foote and finishing at the knee, not forgetting a little bolster under the varicose veine."

James Gibbons Huneker in *Old Fogy* pointed out that prejudices "swell like varicose veins." There is, of course, no room for prejudice in the management of these pervasive pathologic entities. Just as veins have received the attention of poets and are extensively referred to throughout Shakespeare's plays ("stuffed within his bloody veins") while "arteries" are rarely mentioned, they demand the continued attention of surgeons. Since the "improper selection of one's grandparents" that Osler regarded as a major etiologic factor cannot be rectified, we can look forward to a continuous chronology of historical events related to these visible vessels.

Swollen Rivulets

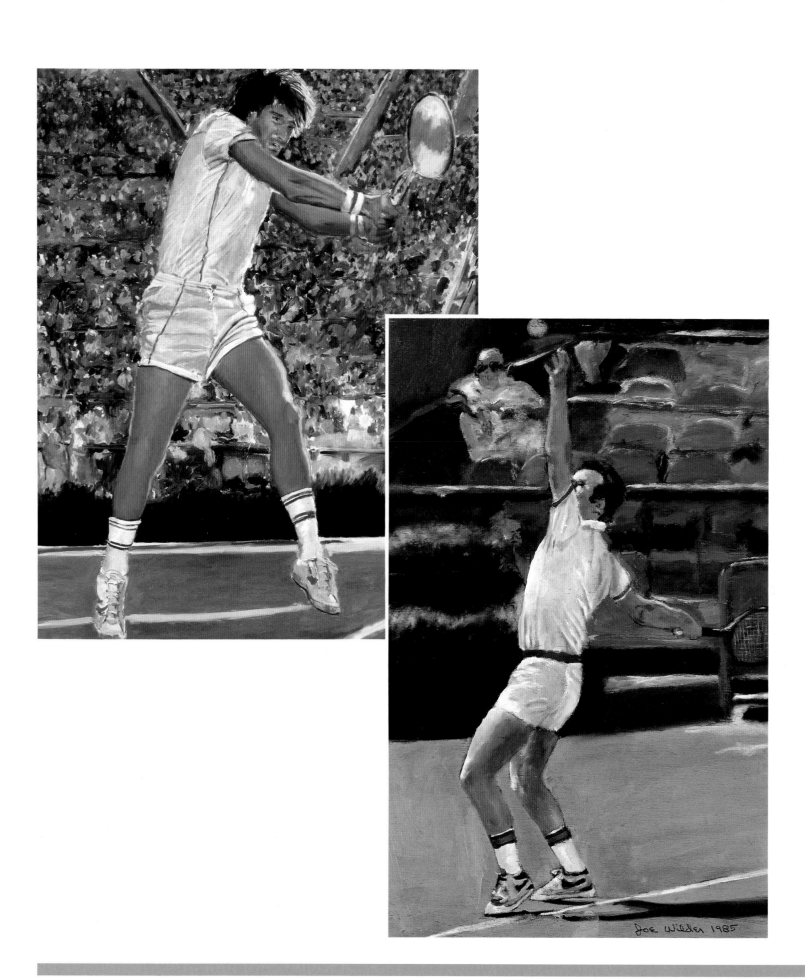

Connors. 1986. Oil on canvas, 36 x 32″. Collection Equitable Life Assurance Society of the United States.
McEnroe. 1986. Oil on board, 18 x 12″.

September 27 is celebrated as the day of martyrdom of the patron saints of surgery, Saints Cosmos and Damian. The twin brothers were famous physicians who accepted no fees and performed many deeds of charity while defending the teachings of Christ. They lived during a period of persecution of Christians and were required to submit to idolatry. When they refused, they were tortured, miraculously saved, but in the year 287 were executed by the sword.

The most famous of their miracles refers to the first "successful" transplantation. Centuries later, according to legend, a devout admirer of the saints was moribund from cancer of his leg. Hoping to be cured, he made a pilgrimage, and after a prayer to the saints, fell asleep in the church. Cosmos and Damian appeared to him in a dream, amputated the diseased leg, and replaced it with the leg of a recently buried Moor. The pilgrim awoke with a viable transplanted black leg; the dead Moor's grave was inspected and contained a diseased white leg. The story brings to mind an old Italian proverb: "If the patient dies, it is the doctor who has killed him, and if he gets well, it is the saints who have cured him."

Perhaps because of this one successful case in the thirteenth century, Cosmos and Damian were selected the patrons of the French Guild of Surgeons. This Guild later became the College of SS Cosmos and Damian. At the time when the faculty of medicine refused to recognize surgery as an academic profession, the College of St. Come (Cosmos) was forced to leave Paris. When surgeons finally were accepted into the faculty of medicine, the School of Medicine actually moved into the buildings of the former College of St. Come.

The legend of the operation was used so often in medieval times that Cosmos and Damian could be considered both the patron saints of the art of surgery and the patron saints of surgery in art. The twin physicians became a recurrent theme in Florentine art in the fifteenth century through the interest of Cosimo Medici, an admirer of their feats. Paintings of the two saints appear on the altar of the cathedral of Florence and throughout the restored monastery of San Marco, where Fra Angelica decorated the walls with scenes from their lives. The great Donatello executed a bas-relief of the saints on the sacristy of San Lorenzo, and Cellini designed a coin on which they are represented. Thus, one of the most modern of our surgical contributions—transplantation—played a major role as a dominant theme of medicine in art more than 500 years ago in medieval days.

Twin Patrons of Two Art Forms

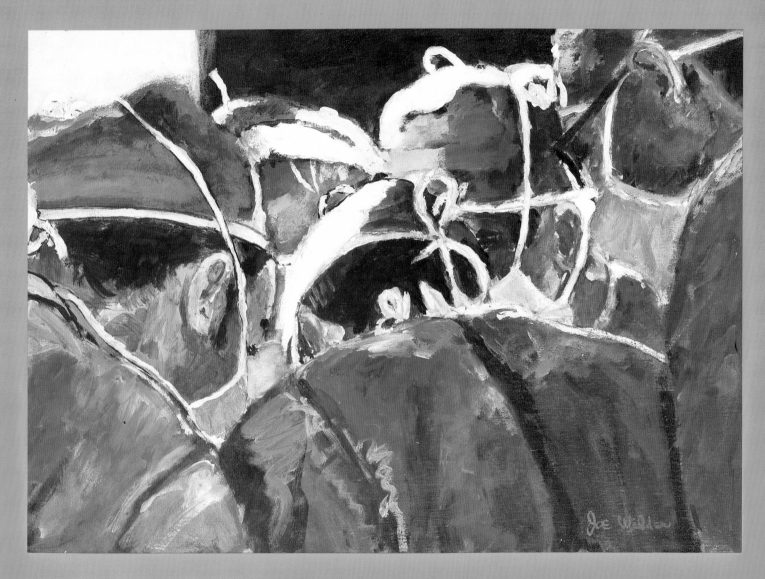

PART SEVEN

Communication

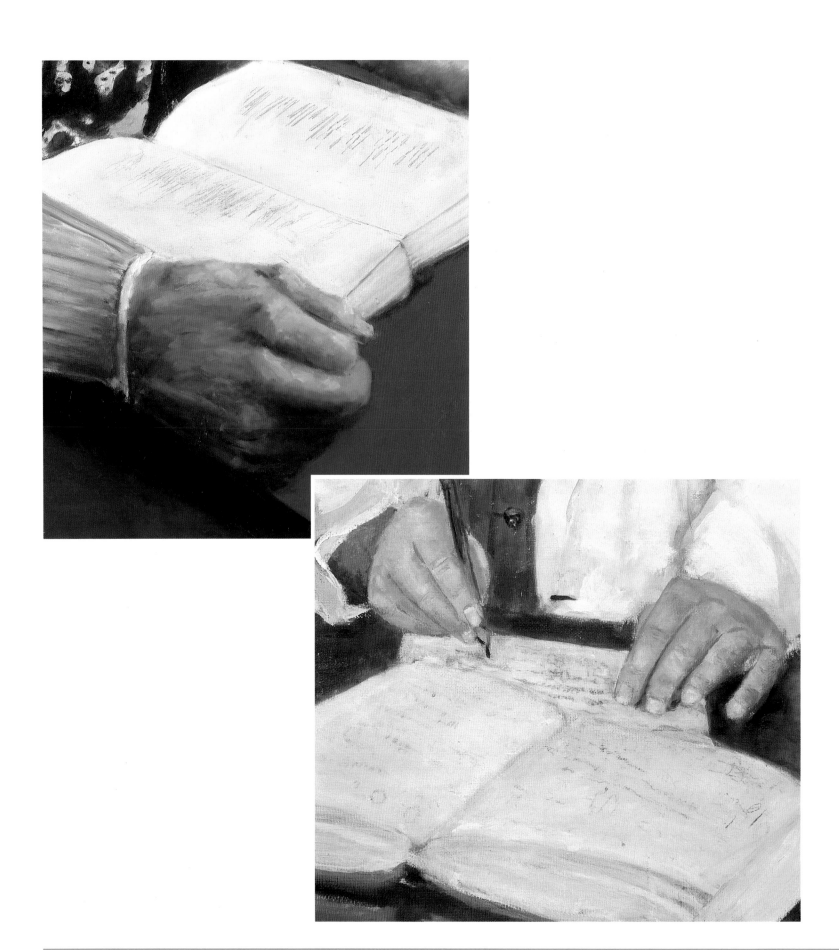

Detail of Luria. 1984 (book and hand).   *Detail of Domagk*. 1987 (hand writing).

I have always felt compelled to write and to contribute to the literature. Part of the stimulus for writing relates to the dissemination of information—whether from experiment or clinical experience. As John Abernathy, the immediate successor to John Hunter, said in the preface to his surgical and physiologic works, published in the early nineteenth century, "Various advantages result even from the publication of opinions; for though we are liable to errors in forming them, yet their promulgation, by exciting investigation and pointing out the deficiencies of our information, cannot be otherwise than useful in the promotion of our science."

I would like to focus on another stimulus to writing, however; one that provides personal reward. It is written in the Book of Job, "Oh that my words were now written! Oh that they were printed in a book!" How often have we wished that we could recapture a thought or a statement that we made? Writing, putting the words down on paper, provides that opportunity. Writing disciplines the thought process, and, at the same time, permits reflective analysis as the thought flows from the "little gray cells" of Agatha Christie's Hercule Poirot to pen or print. Writing necessitates an ultimate refinement of one's thoughts because it imposes on those thoughts a stamp of permanence. The printed word reduces equivocation and presents the thought nakedly exposed, available for use as argument or as the subject of criticism.

Descartes wrote, *"Cogito, ergo sum"*—I think, therefore I am. I write to clarify my thoughts, to impose a period of reflection so that the statement made is the one that I truly want made. It is for this reason that I would personally expand the Cartesian statement to read, *"Scribo ergo cogito ergo sum."* Writing requires an augmentation of thinking. This thesis was synthesized in one line by Francis Bacon: "Reading maketh a full man, conference a ready man, and writing an exact man."

Scribo . . .
Ergo Sum

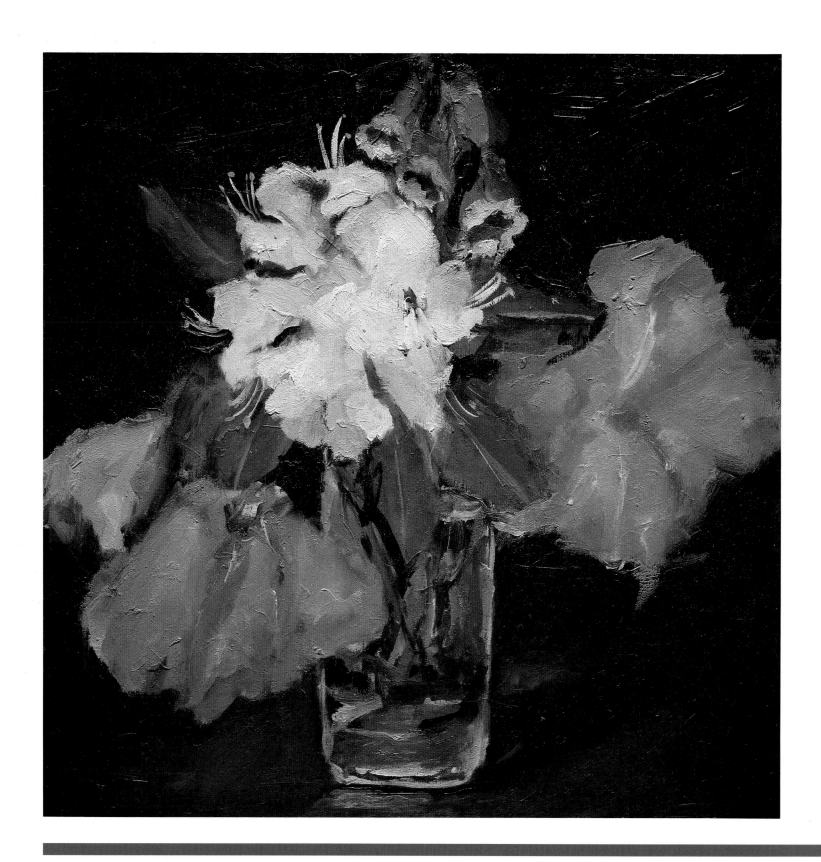

Two Irises, Rhododendron, and Canterbury Bells. 1990. Oil on panel, 12 x 12″. Private collection.

*C*ertainly there are historical precedents for the importance of contributions of relatively youthful surgeons. Andreas Vesalius was 28 when *De Humani Corporis Fabrica* was published in 1543. In 1848, as a 21-year-old student, Henry Gray won the Triennial Prize of the Royal College of Surgeons with a comprehensive survey of the physiology of the nerves associated with vision and eye motion. At age 25 he won the Astley Cooper Prize for his paper, "On the Structure and Use of the Spleen." *Anatomy, Descriptive and Surgical* was published when he was 32, just 2 years before his death from smallpox.

Theodor Billroth's first monograph, "Historical Studies on the Nature and Treatment of Gunshot Wounds From the Fifteenth Century to the Present Time," was published when he was 30; this text advised surgeons to "become familiar not only with teaching but writing." Kaznelson was a senior medical student in Prague when he suggested splenectomy for thrombocytopenia. Michel de Montaigne, in the sixteenth century, emphasized the contributions of youth when he wrote,

> If I were to enumerate all the beautiful human actions, of whatever kind, that have come to my knowledge, I should think I would find that the greater part were performed, both in ancient times and in our own, before the age of thirty, rather than after. Yes, often even in the lives of the same men.

Writing and communicating are important to the role of the physician and surgeon. Henri de Mondeville, who was the first native Frenchman to write a surgical textbook, addressed this issue in the thirteenth century with his statement, "If we know of things unknown at the time of Galen, it is our duty to tell of them in our writings." A quotation that should be taken to heart is that of Sir William Osler, who wrote, "Always note and record the unusual. Keep and compare your observations. Communicate or publish short notes on anything that is striking or new."

Conducting research on a subject, synthesizing the concept, and lucidly expressing thoughts provide a service for a readership, but it is always the author who is the major beneficiary. It is hoped by all interested in education that medical students and residents, despite extreme demands, will pursue personal inquiry and find the time to disseminate the results of their discoveries, however minor they seem. As John Masefield, the Poet Laureate, wrote:

> Adventure on, for from the tiniest clue
> Has come whatever worth man ever knew;
> The next to lighten all men may be you.

Enlightenment

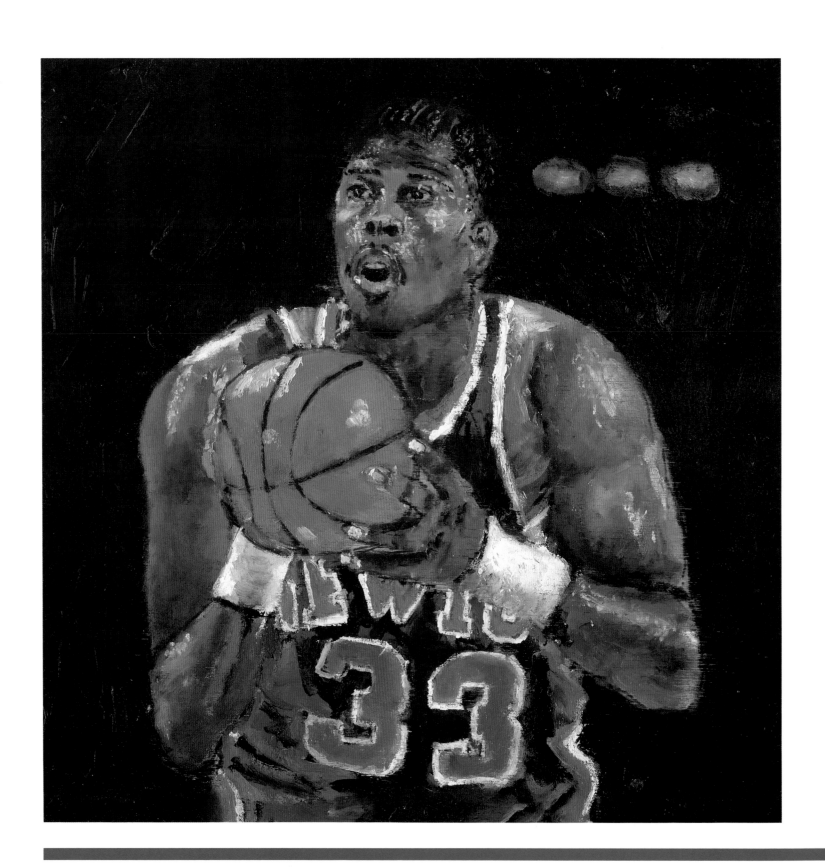

Patrick Ewing. 1990. Oil on panel, 12 x 12″.

On March 7, 1515, St. Thomas Aquinas day, the degree of Doctor in Surgery was conferred in Padua for the first time on a surgeon who did not know Latin. The writings of Lanfranc and Guy de Chauliac appeared in French editions, but the first major original work in surgery to appear in a common or "vulgar" language is credited to Ambroise Paré. It was believed at the time that medicine and surgery would be denigrated by allowing communication to occur in the language of the masses. Voltaire, critical of the use of classical languages for communication about common disorders, cynically wrote, "It is wise to quote that which one does not understand at all in the language one comprehends the least." In the practice of medicine, we are no longer encumbered in our use of language but we still have a linguistic obligation.

The choice of the right word, correctly spelled, in a grammatically acceptable sentence is characteristic of a precise personality, that which is generally demanded of a surgeon. The surgeon who provides an example by correctly spelling "pruritus" and "guaiac," the two most commonly misspelled medical terms, is paying homage to an important feature in the care of the patient, an organ of communication, the records of care. The surgeon who insists that the noun "none" be followed by a singular verb and that "data" be followed by the plural form presents precision that should characterize a surgeon.

It is true that an error in spelling, or syntax, or even a malapropism in no way compromises the care of a patient, but preciseness in diagnosis, management, and technique is so essential that it should also characterize methods of communication.

The choice of words is even more important. Sir William Gull, in his *Study of Medicine,* focused on the importance of the word when he stated, "A word rightly imposed is a landmark indicating so much recovered from the region of ignorance."

In the eighteenth century, Latin lost its role as the vehicle by which the learned communicated their discoveries. English is currently the international language of scientific communication. It is "vulgar" in its true meaning, "spoken by the masses." The scientific and medical communities have grown to the extent of being "masses" in themselves. As long as we invoke a given language to convey important and at times vital thoughts, that language should be treated with appropriate respect and should be used thoughtfully.

Petition for Precise Prose

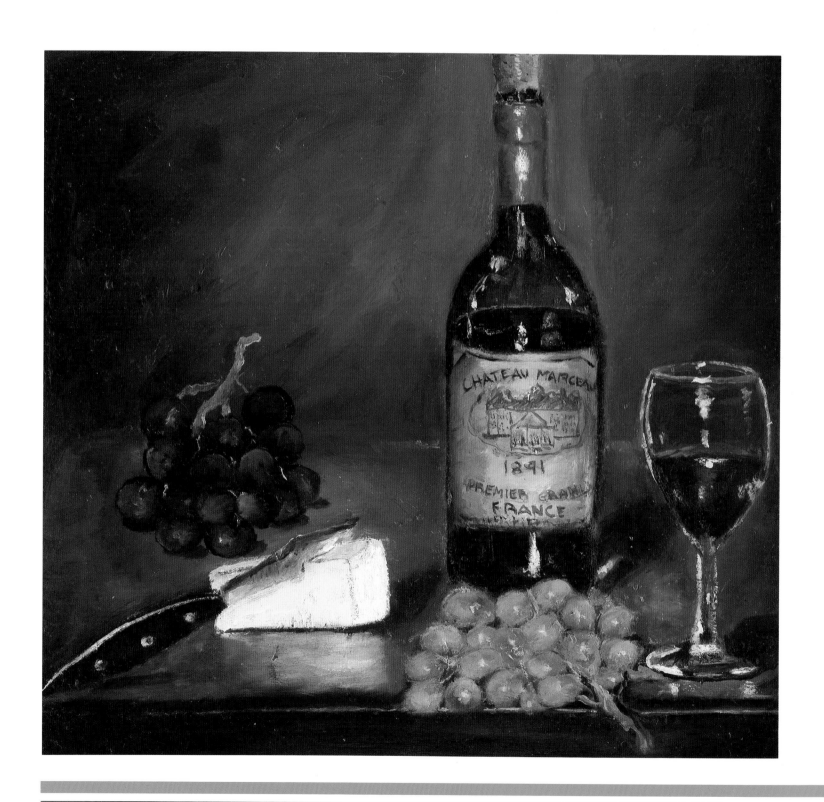

Bottle of Wine, Glass of Wine, Cheese and Grapes. 1988. Oil on panel, 12 x 12″. Collection Mr. and Mrs. Daniel Rose.

In 1863 the *Chicago Times* ran an editorial that read, "The cheek of every American must tingle with shame as he reads the silly, flat and dishwashery utterances of the man who had to be pointed out to intelligent foreigners as the President of the United States." This represented critical comment on Lincoln's memorable Gettysburg address.

Certainly it is easy to recount adverse comments about many if not most of the profound statements made by our surgical progenitors. Witness the derisive statement that appeared in 1825: "We entirely disbelieve that it has ever been performed with success, nor do we think it ever will," relating to the heroic accomplishment of Ephraim McDowell. Similarly, there was a prolonged lack of acceptance with Lord Joseph Lister's introduction of antisepsis.

But criticism remains an important rung on the ladder of knowledge. Satisfying or rebutting that criticism represents an integral step in establishing the permanent value of a concept or a procedure. It is easy for us to be critical; it is difficult to be appropriately critical. Louis Pasteur, with avant garde thought, said, "Little tolerant of frivolous or prejudiced contradiction, contemptuous of that ignorant criticism which doubts on principle, I welcome with open arms the militant attack which has a method in doubting and whose rule of conduct has the motto 'more light'."

Regarding criticism from another vantage point, we can consider every new discovery or application a criticism of things as they are. As W.I.B. Beveridge wrote in *The Art of Scientific Investigation,* "We have to strive to keep our mind receptive, and to examine suggestions made by others fairly and on their own merits, seeking arguments for as well as against them. We must be critical, certainly, but beware lest ideas be rejected because an automatic reaction causes us to see only the arguments against them. We tend especially to resist ideas competing with our own."

Newspaper editorial criticism is featured in a prominent position, while the subsequent retraction appears in small print. In the realm of science, the inappropriate criticism becomes relegated to small print and the affirmation maintains its visibility by becoming a permanent and integral part of our practice.

A Critical Matter

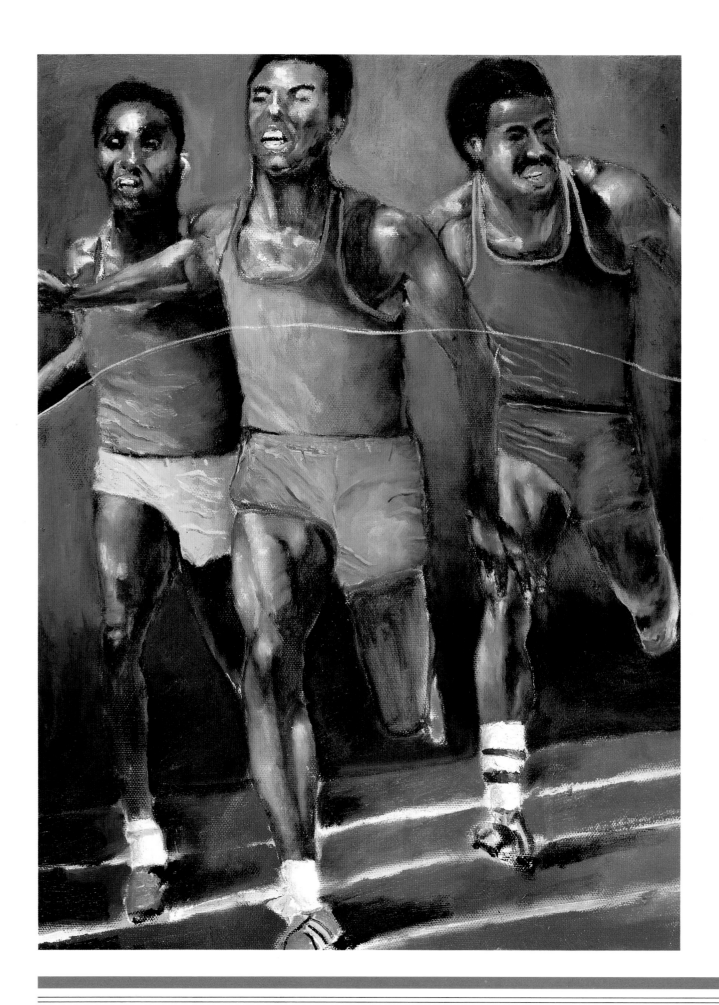

Dead Heat. 1983. Oil on canvas, 17 x 13″.

There is always difficulty in evaluating new scientific discoveries. Abraham Colles' couplet about the attitude of the physician comes to mind: "Wisely suspicious sometimes of the new, Ye give alert acceptance to the true." However, I believe Max Planck was correct when he said a newly revealed scientific truth is accepted not because its opponents become convinced of its validity but because the opponents eventually die and a new generation grows up familiar with it.

Skepticism about new discoveries was also expressed by Leonardo da Vinci in his admonition to "shun the studies in which the results die with the worker." Because the contemporary critic does not have the advantage of knowing what only time can reveal, it is most difficult to assess accurately the value of new findings. It is, therefore, perhaps more appropriate to consider "what's new in surgery?" an expression of the efforts of younger surgeons, with the surgical forum—in accordance with the prescription—providing a podium for displaying their productivity. Consequently, "what's new . . . ?" can also be regarded as "who's new . . . ?" Youth has a distinct advantage. As Claude Bernard stated, "To make discovery, one must be ignorant. Men who have excessive faith in their theories or ideas are not only ill prepared for making discoveries; they also make very poor observations."

Pellegrini cautioned young investigators not to settle for what is measurable instead of pursuing what has not yet been measured. Along similar lines, Jacques Barzun wrote in his *House of Intellect:* "Thousands of young men are at work on little papers; thousands more are racking their brains to think of an experiment to study. Most of them worry more about the acceptability of the subject in the academic eye than about the chances of doing and saying something useful."

Taking all into account, the need for continued interest in research efforts to extend the horizons of surgical science cannot be overemphasized. Its importance is strongly expressed in the letter written in 1775 by John Hunter to Edward Jenner: "I think your solution is just, but why think? Why not try to experiment."

In Search of What's New

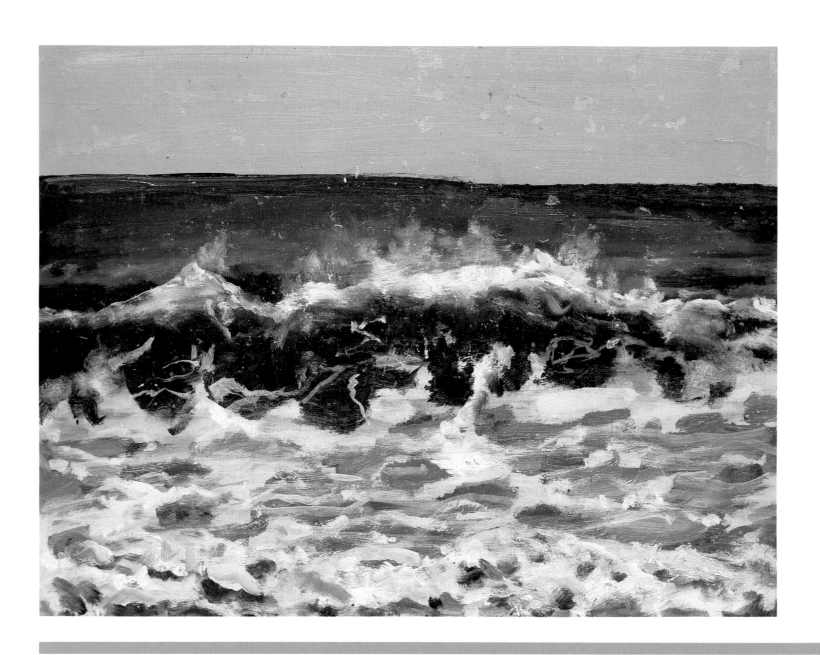

Breaking Waves. 1985. Oil on panel, 10 x 12″.

My personal thesis is that surgical judgment should be based on "numbers," with the caveat that the numbers themselves may be suspect. The numeric facts then form the basis for algorithms, which are defined as sets of rules for solving a problem in a finite number of steps.

Certainly, there is little question that the way to truth is the minute examination of facts, and some facts must be expressed as specific numbers. In the eighteenth century Robert Burns, the Scottish poet, wrote, "Facts are chiels that winna ding, an' downa be disputed." (Facts are entities that cannot be manipulated or disputed.) For surgeons, data must stand out as roadmaps to paths of therapy that their own emotions or visceral reaction would like to traverse during their care of patients.

The advantage of quantification has been long appreciated: witness Francis Bacon's statement at the turn of the eighteenth century: "As Physic advances farther and farther . . . it will require fresh assistance from Mathematics." However, this attitude can be countered by a realization that a mathematic expression does not necessarily mean truth and may only add arrogance to error.

Facts cannot stand alone; they must be entered into our natural "computers," and synapsed in a logical fashion. As Aldous Huxley wrote, "Facts are ventriloquists' dummies. Sitting on a wise man's knee they may be made to utter words of wisdom; elsewhere, they say nothing, or talk nonsense." A famous physician, speaking through his prime character, Sherlock Holmes, uttered a note of caution regarding the isolated fact. "From a drop of water a logician could infer the possibility of an Atlantic or Niagara. . . ." Data remain the unequivocal desiderata on which clinical judgments must be based. Numbers are the nuclei from which the logical thoughts can emanate in pseudopodal patterns.

A Nucleus of Numbers

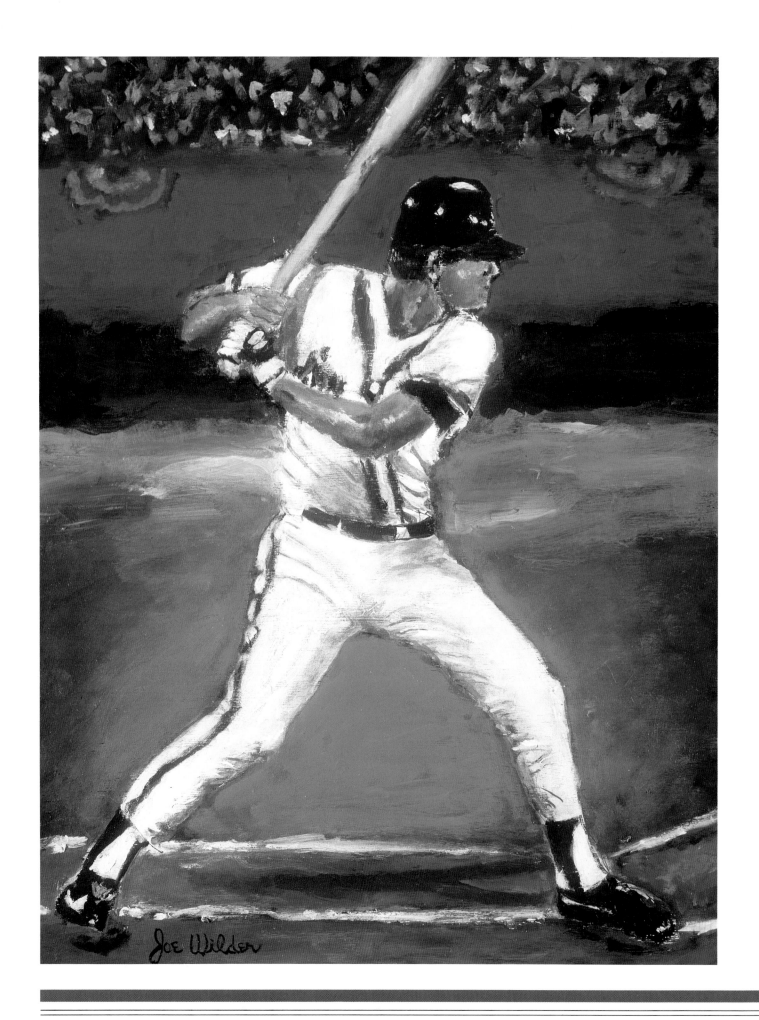

Dale Murphy. 1989. Oil on panel, 17 x 13″.

Medical record keeping has long been a focus of concentration. In 1752, at the inception of the oldest hospital in the United States, the Pennsylvania Hospital, it was specified that "practitioners should keep a fair account (in a book provided for that purpose) of the several patients under their care. . . ." Osler emphasized on numerous occasions that medical records are an integral and valuable component of good medical care.

Difficulties related to the keeping of medical records result primarily from the personal disenchantment of the physician with translating thoughts and deeds into written words. Keeping a careful medical record is generally an altruistic action, since it is of greatest benefit to the patient and to future physicians. As Lois DeBakey pointed out: "There is a cavalier attitude toward verbal expression. While research is vigorously pursued in methods of storing and retrieving information by computers, the communication of an idea undistorted from one mind to another continues to be neglected."

Illegibility frequently compounds the problem of disregard for maintaining a permanent record. It is amazing to note that the same hand that is direct and neat with a scalpel becomes paralytic or dyskinetic with a pen.

Medical school curriculums and residency programs need to stress the importance of the record as an instrument of communication. Its role in the care of an individual patient must be pointed out, as must the fact that it is the main legal document relating to the patient's progress. Furthermore, training programs must emphasize the record's function of providing the cumulative data on which generalized scientific conclusions can be based.

Appreciation of record-oriented problems necessitates major efforts to avoid three ills: (1) *ill*egibility, (2) anything that could be interpreted as *ill*egality, and (3) precise verbal definition rather than relative *ill*iteracy.

Reckoning With Records

173

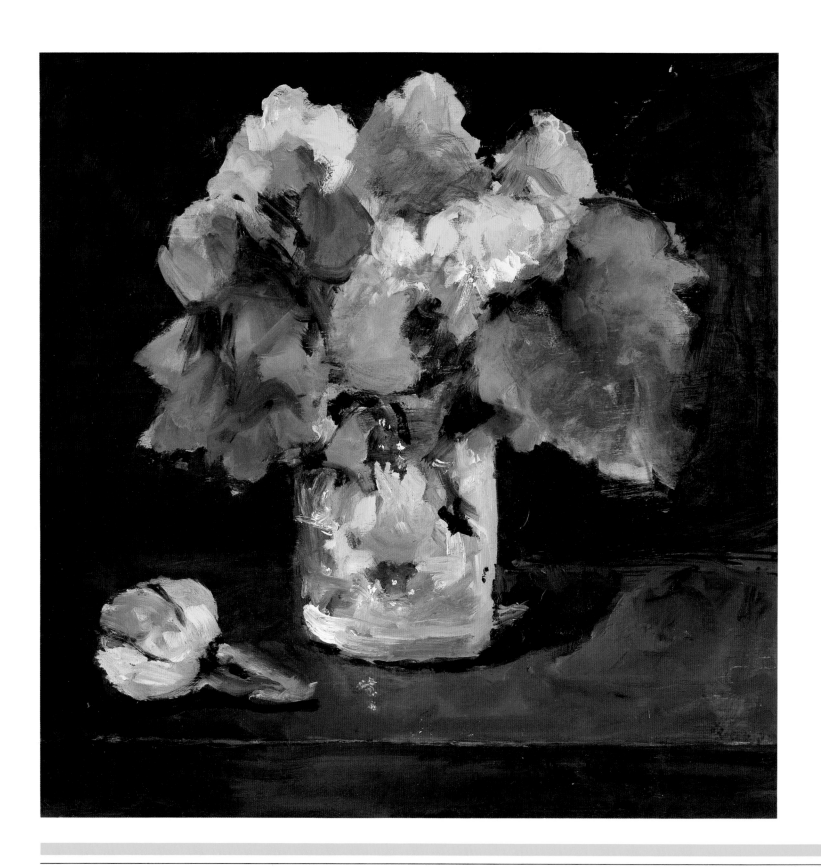

Maple Tulips. 1992. Oil on panel, 13 x 13″.

*B*eware the ides of March," the soothsayer warned Julius Caesar. This warning is also an implicit prognostication.

Warnings and prognostications are also part of the dialogue of a surgeon. We warn against smoking, dietary indiscretions, and excessive intake of alcohol; all too frequently the words are heard but not heeded. John Ring's eighteenth century treatise on gout could well apply to the response to the Surgeon General's statement on smoking: "The still voice of reason is not heard; the sober dictates of discretion are disregarded and the friendly warnings of the physician are either totally forgotten or treated with ridicule and contempt." Samuel Johnson said it succinctly: "Among the innumerable follies by which we lay up in our youth . . . there is scarce any against which warnings are of less efficacy, than the neglect of health."

While warnings often fall on deaf ears, our medical prognostications are digested, ruminated on, and recalled repeatedly. Guy de Chauliac, in the fourteenth century, emphasized that the surgeon should be cautious in prognostications. In *Ars Chirurgica*, he wrote that a surgeon "ought to be gracious to the sick, considerate to his associates, cautious in his prognostications." The late, great cancer surgeon, George Pack, simply stated an important truth: "The patient's family will never forgive a guarantee of cure that failed and the patient will not let the physician forget a pronouncement of incurability if he is so fortunate as to survive."

A surgeon's statement may be as irrevocable as the incision, and although verbal repair and remodeling may be attempted, a permanent impression (scar) persists. As the March Hare admonished, "You should say what you mean"—but with caution.

Warnings and Prognostications

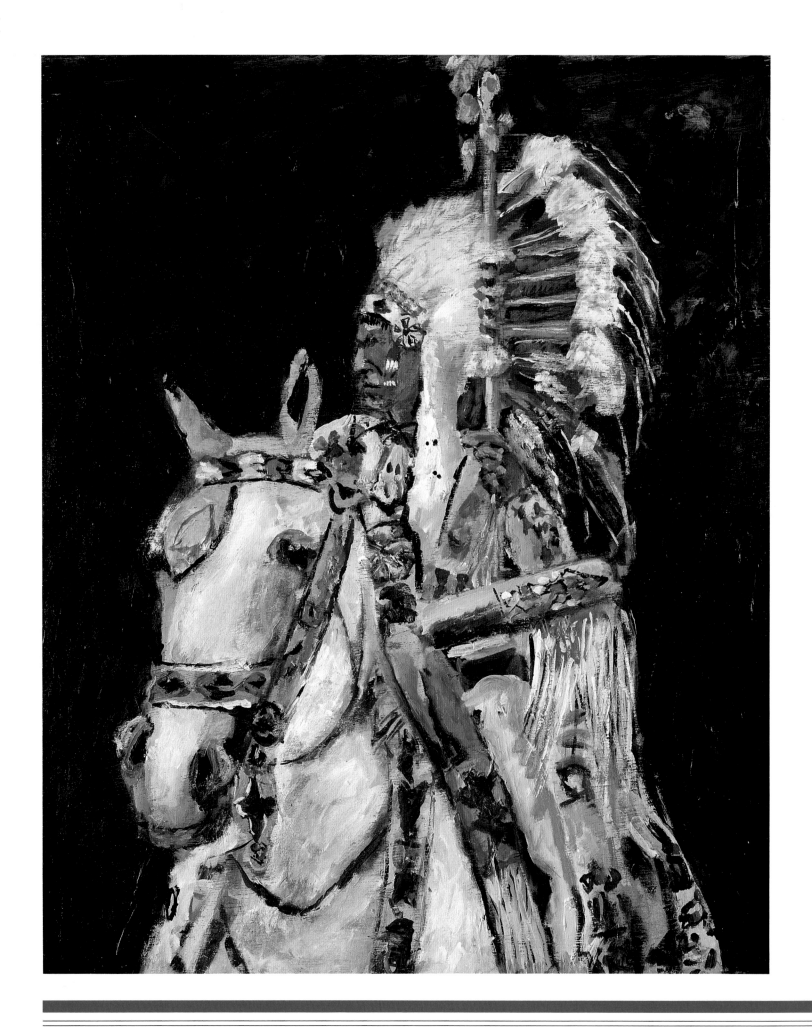

Native American. 1991. Oil on panel, 28 x 20″.

Amerigo Vespucci is representative of the leading role played by Italy in expanding the world during the end of the fifteenth and the beginning of the sixteenth centuries. Cristoforo Colombo (Columbus), Giovanni Caboto (Cabot) of Genoa, and Giovanni da Verrazzano, along with Vespucci of Firenze, were all primary figures at the time.

A vignette about the naming of our land is timely. In 1507, a German mapmaker produced the first printed map of America, also the first map to include the name America (albeit on the southern half of the hemisphere). In a book that this mapmaker published that same year, he wrote:

> I do not see why anyone would rightly forbid naming it Amerige—land of Americus, as it was, after its discoverer Americus, a man of acute genius—or America, since both Europe and Asia have received their names from women.

Later, the same cartographer, deciding that Vespucci did not rightly deserve the honor, deleted "America" from his subsequent maps, but the name has persisted.

This same period also saw significant Italian contributions to surgery. The first surgical compendium, *Chirurgia Parva*, by Guy de Chauliac, was issued in 1490 in Venice. Leonardo da Vinci (1452-1519) added to our knowledge of anatomy. The *Practica Copiosa* of Giovanni da Vigo (1460-1525), which dealt with wounds from firearms, went through 52 editions. Bartolomomeo Maggi championed Ambroise Paré's cause and carried out experiments to prove that gunshot wounds were neither burned nor poisonous. But the most memorable Italian surgeon was Gasparo Tagliacozzi (1546-1599) of Bologna, who revived the operation of rhinoplasty. Like Vespucci, he was dishonored and held in disrepute by Paré and others; his operation was regarded as meddling with the handiwork of God. Tagliacozzi's remains were exhumed and buried in unconsecrated ground. But he lives on today and is generally regarded as the Father of Plastic Surgery.

In this parallelism between geography and surgery in sixteenth century Italy, we have two who made contributions, who were the object of erasures, and who have survived with repute in our time. We have examples of the rebirth of the reputations of two who lived during an era of intellectual rebirth, the Renaissance.

Italian Influence and Irrepressibility

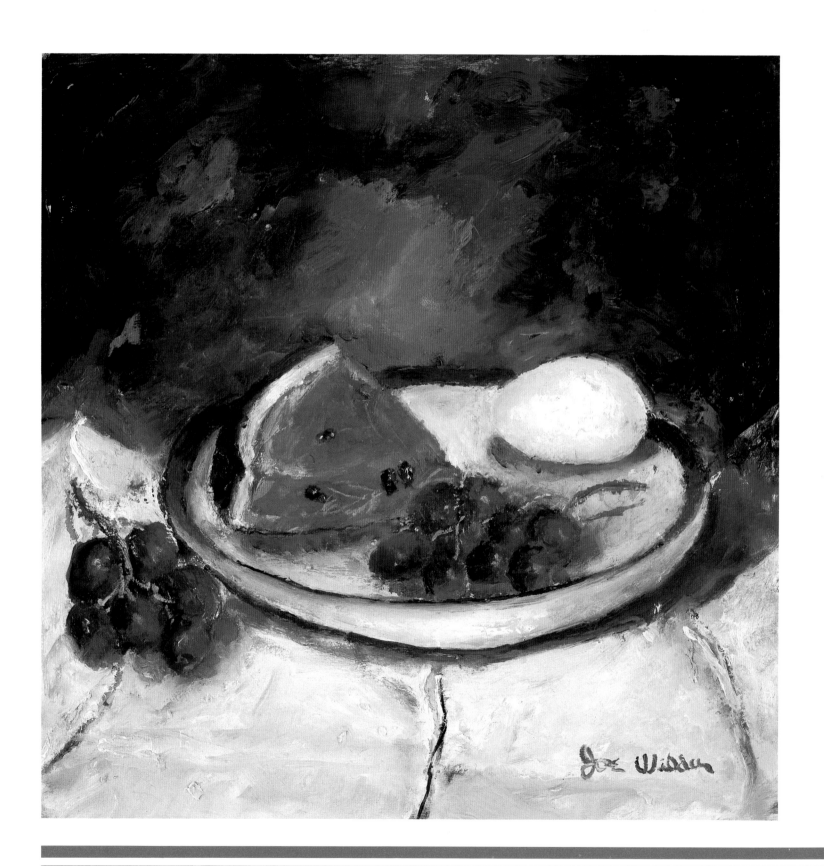

Watermelon, Red Grapes, and One White Egg. 1991. Oil on panel, 12 x 12″.

William Shakespeare's plays contain more than 450 major medical references, often used to illustrate a point. The great Bard expressed the medical knowledge of the average literate man of the day. "The nimble spirits in the arteries" (*Love's Labour's Lost*) alludes to the pre-Harvey theory that the arteries contained air and not blood.

Shakespeare's reference to matters surgical were few and essentially focused on wounds. Elizabethan surgeons were restricted by law from giving any internal medicines, even to cure external injuries. As Wells wrote describing the rules made by Harvey for the house officers at St. Bartholomew's, "The doctor's treatment of the poor chirurgeons in these rules is sufficiently despotic . . . but the chirurgeons in their acquiesence showed that they merited no better handling."

In Elizabethan life the management of wounds was a common medical experience, and Shakespeare's observant eye records many views regarding therapy. Corrosives were applied to serious and dangerous wounds: "Though parting be a fretful corrosive, It is applied to a deathful wound" (*Henry VI*). Balsam was also used on wounds: "Is this the balsam that the usurping senate pours into captain's wounds?" (*Timon of Athens*), as were plasters: "You rub the sore when you should bring the plaster" (*The Tempest*). One of the interesting methods of managing wounds involved a roll of lint or flax that was thrust into the deep wound to control bleeding. This was known as a "tent," and knowledge of this meaning is necessary to appreciate "but modest doubt is call'd the beacon of the wise, the tent that searches to th' bottom of the worst" (*Troilus and Cressida*). Hemorrhage from wounds was of major concern, and there were few effective ways of controlling it, although ligature, cautery, and pressure had all been tried. Control of hemorrhage was the surgeon's domain, as indicated by Portia in her famous cornering of Shylock: "Have by some surgeon, Shylock, on your charge, To stop his wounds lest he do bleed to death" (*Merchant of Venice*). Two of the household medicines used in Shakespeare's time to control bleeding are mentioned in his works. "I'll fetch some *flax* and *white of egg* To apply to his bleeding face" (*King Lear*), and "I shall desire you of more acquaintance, good Master *Cobweb*, If I cut my finger I shall make bold with you" (*Midsummer Night's Dream*). It was appreciated that wounds healed slowly, as stated by Iago, "What wound did heal but by degrees?" (*Othello*)

But my extraction of quotes for a surgical audience is an extreme disservice. As Samuel Johnson wrote in his preface to a 1765 edition of Shakespeare's works, "He that tries to recommend him by select quotations will succeed like the pedant in Hierocles, who, when he offered his house to sale, carried a brick in his pocket as a specimen."

Shakespeare and Surgery

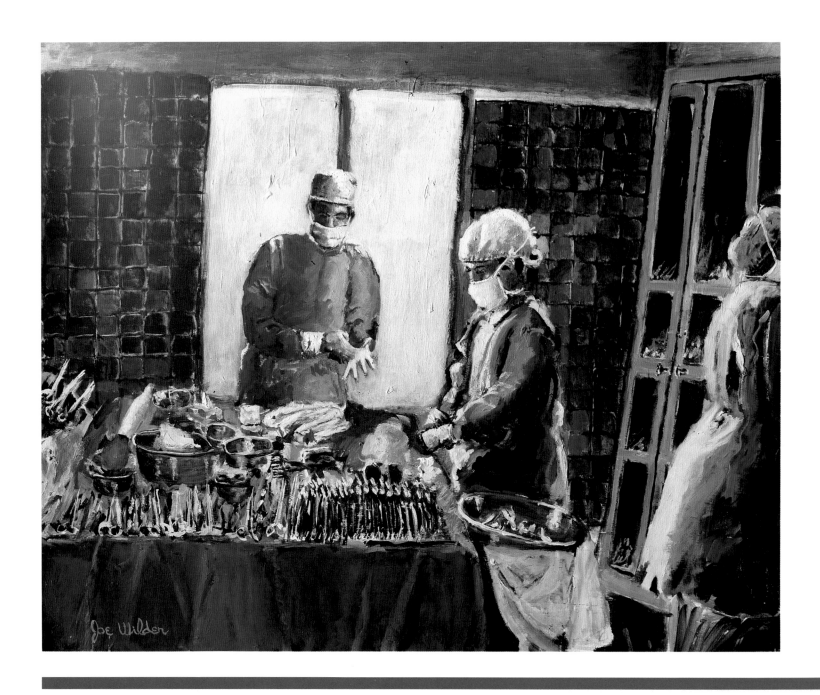

Checking Instruments. 1989. Oil on panel, 13 x 18″.

As I mused over a drawing of Péan by Toulouse-Lautrec, I reflected that more people, and even more surgeons, would recognize the name of the artist more than that of the man who is credited with priority in the development and use of a hemostatic forceps. Honoré de Balzac wrote, "The glory of surgeons is like that of actors, who exist only in their lifetime and whose talent is no longer appreciable once they have disappeared."

In Hippocrates' famous statement, "Life is short and the art is long," art referred specifically to medicine. But the sequence and comparison could be used to show that the physician or surgeon, who contributes to the preservation of life, has but a brief span as the focus of attention or as the object of recognition, while the artist, whose product potentially affords pleasure for posterity, maintains a permanent notability. Even the lesser artist, Henri Gervex, who also painted a portrait of Péan ("Avant l'Opération"), remains better known to the French than does his surgical subject.

Matisse had a cancer of the colon removed by three famous French surgeons, including Rene Leriche, who became the subject of a lithograph by the impressionist. How many can speak to the accomplishments of the surgeon of eponymic proportion? In England, the name of Sir Joshua Reynolds retains a luminescence even greater than that of his famous subject, John Hunter. It was from the Reynolds portrait that William Sharp produced the engraving of the eminent surgeon seated at a table preparing a manuscript, a work considered by art critics to be one of the foremost portraits in English art.

Most British and many Americans are devotees of the caricaturist, Spy, but how many remember his surgical subject, Sir Henry Thompson, who had the distinction of operating on two emperors, Leopold I of Belgium and Napoleon III of France, for bladder stone? To enforce the issue on our own home ground, compare the recognition of the names of the artist Thomas Eakins and two of his subjects, Dr. D. Hayes Agnew, professor of surgery at the University of Pennsylvania, and Dr. Samuel Gross, professor of surgery at Jefferson Medical College in Philadelphia and first president of the American Surgical Association.

Joseph Conrad wrote, "The artist appeals to that part of our being which is not dependent on wisdom; to that in us which is a gift and not an acquisition and therefore, more permanently endearing." As Havelock Ellis wrote, "The artist writes his own autobiography," but for the surgeon, the quotation of Ramón y Cajal is perhaps the most pertinent: "Glory is nothing more than oblivion postponed."

Cures Have No Curators

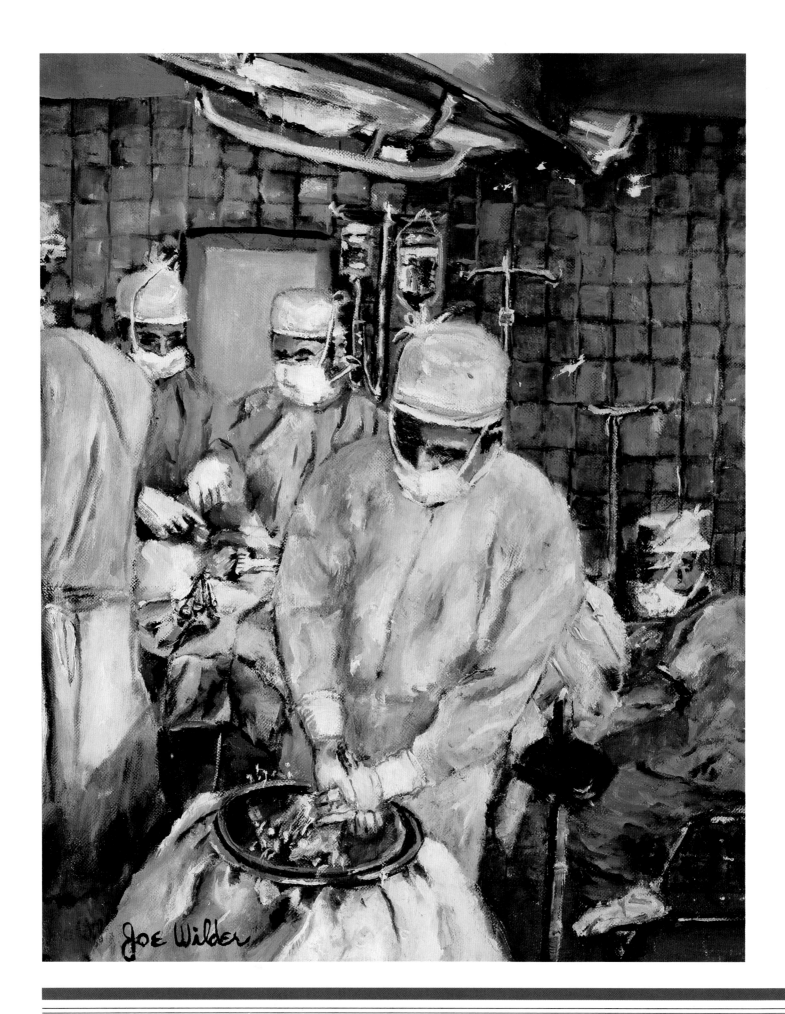

Surgeons at Work. 1987. Oil on canvas, 14 x 11″. Collection Nick Wilder.

Dr. Joe Wilder's rendition of *Surgeons at Work* is an example showing a subject that has captured artists' attention for centuries. I am reminded of two more critical sixteenth century Dutch etchings with the same title. Lucas van Leyden depicted a surgeon seated in a chair performing a minor operation on the ear of a stoic peasant who was seated on the floor. Symbolism permeates the work. The surgeon's costume defines a charlatan; the large purse that he wears stresses that his goal is monetary compensation. The stone under the patient's left hand suggests that the procedure is unnecessary; the removal of stones a folly, or stupidity. In the same genre, Cornelis Dusart etched a village surgeon lancing the arm of an agonized patient. The surgeon's hood contains a barber's razor, and on the wall is a forceps for extracting teeth.

More modern artistic interpretations of the surgeon have been less deprecating. One could look to works by Sir Joshua Reynolds, Toulouse-Lautrec, Henri Matisse, Thomas Eakins, and George Bellows to prove this point. An empathy and sense of camaraderie should underscore the artist's representation of the modern surgeon who is an artist in depth. Dana Atchley wrote, "Like all great art, the art of medicine is the skillful and creative application of a scientific discipline to a human problem."

The art of medicine emphasizes the conjectural; the art of surgery begins with the conjectural and proceeds with the goal of being effectual. Surgery is analogous to an artist's restoration of a piece of art that was produced in the past. Based on a scientific appreciation of normal anatomy and physiology of the human canvas and a recognition of the deterioration or disorder that requires repair, the surgeon applies a personal artistry that has evolved from a primitive period through a classical period to the present period of dynamic modernism.

Sir Berkeley Moynihan poignantly focused on the artistry of surgery: "As art surgery is incomparable to the beauty of its medium, in its supreme mastery required for its perfect accomplishment, and in the issues of life, suffering, and death, which it so powerfully controls."

Art of an Art